HEALTH AND WELL-BEING FOR YOUNG PEOPLE

HEALTH AND WELL-BEING FOR YOUNG PEOPLE

BUILDING RESILIENCE AND EMPOWERMENT

COLIN GOBLE AND NATASHA BYE-BROOKS

BLOOMSBURY ACADEMIC

LONDON • NEW YORK • OXFORD • NEW DELHI • SYDNEY

BLOOMSBURY ACADEMIC
Bloomsbury Publishing Plc
50 Bedford Square, London, WC1B 3DP, UK
1385 Broadway, New York, NY 10018, USA
29 Earlsfort Terrace, Dublin 2, Ireland

BLOOMSBURY, BLOOMSBURY ACADEMIC and the Diana logo are trademarks of Bloomsbury Publishing Plc

First published in Great Britain 2016 by Palgrave
Reprinted by Bloomsbury Academic 2022

A catalogue record for this book is available from the British Library.

A catalog record for this book is available from the Library of Congress.

ISBN: PB: 978-0-230-39026-3

To find out more about our authors and books visit www.bloomsbury.com and sign up for our newsletters.

*The authors would like to dedicate this book to their very own
'young people', Joe and Lewis (Natasha) and Callum and Dylan (Colin).
They have of course taught us more than any book could.*

CONTENTS

ACKNOWLEDGEMENTS

The authors and publisher wish to thank The Tufnell Press for kind permission to reproduce Table 7.1, 'Live births and birth rates...', on page 96.

The authors would like to acknowledge the encouragement and support of our colleagues and students on the BA Childhood, Youth & Community Studies programme at the University of Winchester.

We would also like to acknowledge the support of the team at Palgrave publishers for their patience and professionalism.

1

INTRODUCTION: WHAT ARE THE ISSUES?

This book is about health issues for young people. It is based on a module taught as part of the BA in 'Childhood, Youth & Community Studies' at the University of Winchester. As undergraduate students are wont to, many have asked us if there was a single textbook to which they could refer to provide key reading. Being good educationalists we have always responded by encouraging them to read widely, and to make use of the variety of excellent books, journals and other academic and scientific resources that relate to the various topics addressed in this book. However, we also realized that perhaps they did have a point. The sources we refer students to tend either to not quite cover all the areas or age range required, or, in a rapidly changing policy and research landscape, to be somewhat out of date. So, we felt that it would indeed be useful to have a book that addresses two main aims. First, to introduce and outline the general topic area of health and well-being for young people, including key concepts, historical and theoretical perspectives. And second, to identify the key issues and debates that relate to the health and well-being of young people in the UK (and more widely) at the present time.

In this opening chapter we begin by first identifying who we are talking about when we use the phrase 'young people'. We will then go on to define what we mean by the terms 'health' and 'well-being', before setting out the main theories and frameworks that inform and underpin our approach to thinking about health issues for young people. This will lead into a discussion of what the main health issues are that will be addressed in subsequent chapters. First, then, what and who do we mean by 'young people'?

Who are we talking about?

Essentially we are talking about people in the life stage commonly described as adolescence. The United Nations (UN) and the World Health Organization (WHO) define adolescence as the period between the ages of 10 and 19. In the UK, however, the government's 'Children and Young People's Health Outcomes

Forum' recommends that for most policy and research purposes adolescence is broken down into the following age bands:

- 10–14 years – referred to as 'early adolescence'
- 15–19 years – referred to as 'late adolescence'
- 20–25 years – referred to as 'young adulthood'

In the UK, there are around 7.4 million young people falling across these age bands, constituting around 12 per cent of the total population (Hagell, Coleman and Brooks, 2013).

Adolescence is most often thought of as a biologically defined life stage. To understand it fully, however, it also needs to be seen as a social and cultural construct. The way we conceive of adolescence at this time, in this society, is very much an embodiment of the current historical and cultural period, and not a fixed and immutable phenomenon. In different cultures, at different periods in history, the life stage that we define as adolescence has not existed in the way that we would recognize it. Young teenage girls, for example, would be, and in parts of the world still are, deemed old enough to marry and begin childbearing; and young teenage boys would be, and still are, deemed old enough to bear arms, or undertake long arduous hours of hard physical work. The nature and experience of adolescence has always been, and remains, subject to change across time and cultures – and within cultures too. This means that, whilst the biological aspects of health and well-being for young people are relatively fixed, the same cannot be said about many of the psycho-social factors. This is reflected in those issues which are seen as particularly significant in relation to the health and well-being of young people.

Defining health and well-being

Ideas of 'health' and 'well-being' can vary widely, and are shaped by a variety of factors. Ewles and Simnett (2003) identify the importance of our direct experiences, usually of ill health in ourselves and/or people close to us, in shaping what we know. We also accumulate knowledge about health from a variety of sources, including 'official' health education and promotion sources, TV dramas and documentaries, media and news reports, and what might be called 'folk sources' – including knowledge passed down by word of mouth in schools, workplaces, pubs, etc.; and nowadays, increasingly via social media and the internet.

Our understanding of health is also shaped by our ethical beliefs and values. 'Health' is regarded as a positive value in Western culture and, increasingly, as the 'reward' for living a healthy lifestyle – eating the right things, doing the right amount of exercise, practising 'safe sex', drinking alcohol in moderation and not smoking or taking drugs. This also suggests that moral judgements may be made about those who experience ill health as a result of not adhering to such a lifestyle – as distinct from just 'bad luck'. Implied here then is a distinction between the 'deserving' and 'undeserving' that can become a significant factor in debates about the allocation of resources – to treat drug addicts, for example.

Our understanding of health is also shaped to some extent by our expectations. In modern, affluent societies we have come to expect a long and generally healthy life, with odd interludes perhaps of ill health that are 'cured', or at least mitigated in their effects, by medical interventions and health treatments. We have been encouraged to become 'consumers' of health services, and to expect a pill, a treatment or a cure for whatever health problem we face.

Defining health and well-being, then, is not quite as straightforward as it may at first seem. A useful place to begin, however, is with the classic WHO definition from its early, aspirational, post-Second World War period, which defines health as:

> A state of complete physical, mental and social well-being, not merely the absence of disease and infirmity.
>
> (WHO, 1946)

Today this definition appears simplistic, but it does have the merits of including mental and social, as well as physiological, dimensions of health, and of conceptualizing health as a positive concept underpinning well-being, rather than just a state of freedom from illness and impairment. This positive aspect was elaborated upon further in a later WHO definition which highlighted the interplay between individuals, groups and the surrounding environment – physical, psychological and cultural:

> ......the extent to which an individual or group is able, on the one hand, to realise aspirations and satisfy needs; and on the other hand to change or cope with the environment. Health is, therefore, seen as a resource for everyday life, not the object of living; it is a positive concept emphasizing social and personal resources, as well as physical capabilities. (WHO, 1984)

This conceptualization emphasizes to an even greater extent the multidimensional nature of health and well-being, including:

● **Physical health and well-being** – as in a healthy development and functioning of the body, although not necessarily conforming to the relatively narrow range of physical normality that biomedical approaches have often worked to. This is an important point when we come to look at the impact of living with physical, sensory or intellectual impairment for example.

- *Mental and emotional health and well-being* – as in a healthy functioning of the mind, although, again, we would argue that this requires going some way beyond where conventional biomedical approaches might currently draw the line of 'normality', embracing as we do the concept of 'neurodiversity' (Silberman, 2015).

- *Spiritual health and well-being* – here, we mean not only an attachment or adherence to a particular religious faith or philosophy (although this may well be a factor for some people), but rather a sense of meaning and purpose in life, which acts both as a foundation and a motivator for an active engagement with the world. As well as the traditional religions, examples here might include things like political activism to improve social justice or the environment, or a desire to seek personal fulfilment through a particular career, sport or unpaid interest – and, of course, a simple desire to achieve happiness and well-being in personal relationships and day-to-day life.

- *Social health and well-being* – as in the interrelationship between the individual and social and cultural environment they inhabit, including political, ideological and economic factors that may impact on them.

Our intention is to address all of these dimensions of health and well-being in our subsequent discussions, underpinning our approach with a combination of **'holistic'**, **'humanistic'** and **'ecological'** conceptions of health and well-being.

By **'holistic'** we mean a conception of health and well-being that recognizes the importance of all of the dimensions identified above, not as separate and mutually exclusive, but as interacting influences. By **'humanistic'** we mean a conception that highlights the value of the individual, and a 'person-centred' ethos that recognizes that, whatever the commonalities of the issues and experiences young people face, emphasis should always be given to empowering individuals to find solutions that meet their own needs, goals and aspirations. And by **'ecological'** we mean the recognition that all individuals sit within complex webs of interrelationships and interactions with their environment – physical, psychological and sociocultural – and that the impact and influence of these environmental factors are highly significant for their health and well-being.

Much of the above discussion could apply to any age group. Focusing as we are, however, on young people, we are particularly concerned to recognize what is specific to them. The dramatic physiological and psychological changes that the adolescent life stage involves mean that this is almost inevitably a time of significant change, and, perhaps, some turmoil for most young people. For many, this will not turn into anything more sinister than transient spells of grumpiness, moodiness and some arguments with parents and/or carers as boundaries and relationships are reshaped and redefined. For some, however, it can lead to serious and sometimes devastating problems which can affect their health and well-being for the remainder of their adult lives, and even seriously shorten their adult lifespan.

We don't, however, want to set this book up with too negative a premise. Health and well-being are, after all, positive concepts, and it is a contention of the authors that the aim of any rational approach to public health should be to identify those factors that promote positive health and well-being for young people, and to base interventions and responses on an evidence-based approach that helps to promote those goals. This should help to ensure the greatest possibility of successful health and well-being outcomes for young people, as well as best professional practice, whilst also pointing us towards the best use of resources.

An evidence-based approach to health promotion strategy, policy and service delivery for young people, at both national and local levels, may sound perfectly logical and rational. Sadly, policy agendas aimed at young people often seem to be far from logical and rational, and frequently seem to be driven by ideological, rather than evidence-based, agendas. This is particularly true in areas such as sexual health and substance misuse, where major controversies around appropriate strategies exist. We will look at some of these debates as we address these topics in later chapters.

Coleman, Hendry and Kleop (2007) point out that young people themselves often have different concerns and ways of thinking about health than adults. Their work shows that many young people tend to think about health primarily in terms of the 'here and now', rather than thinking about distant, future consequences. They may, for example, tend to think about diet and nutrition in terms of its impact on their appearance, and particularly how their peer group may judge them, rather than about any long-term health consequences of obesity such as the development of type 2 diabetes or heart disease in middle age. This has important implications for the nature of health promotion and health education activities aimed at young people, and the implications for this will also be addressed in later chapters.

Ultimately, the aim we most aspire to is to encourage an 'empowering' approach to health promotion and education. By this we mean helping young people to develop the knowledge, skills and confidence they need to make the best decisions about their own health and well-being; to withstand and become resilient to the almost inevitable health-related pressures and risk factors they may face in order to minimize harm and reduce any lasting damage; and, ideally, to demand of adults – including politicians, public services and corporate interests – that they live up to *their* responsibilities to create social, economic and institutional environments that promote, rather than damage, their health and well-being.

This last point brings us to the issue of the 'rights' of children and young people. Space precludes us from too detailed a discussion of children's and young people's rights, but we feel it is important to state from the start that we adhere to the principle embodied in the UN Declaration of the Rights of the Child (1989) that children and young people should enjoy 'special protection' (Principle 1) with particular regard to their health and well-being (Principle 4). These rights have been incorporated into various pieces of legislation and policy in the UK, including the Children's Acts (1989 and 2004), The Human Rights Act (1998), The Disability Discrimination Act (2005), The Children's and Families Act (2014) and The Care Act (2014). These and other pieces of legislation and policy will be referred to as we address each topic area. In line with these principles we would argue that access to good health care, public institutions, practices and policies that promote the optimization of health and well-being in young people is a cornerstone of a modern, civilized society and an important part of the investment that society makes in its young people.

An especially important aim of health promotion effort with young people is the development of their capacity for 'resilience' to health problems and risks. Resilience has become an important part of recent discourse around the health and well-being of children and young people, and we shall refer to it repeatedly in this book. We would like to echo here, however, the concern raised by Coleman and Hagell (2011) that young people's 'resilience' to health problems and risks should not be promoted as a personal or innate quality, but rather something that is acquired with appropriate adult support. It is important that young people are not unfairly exposed to the criticism that they are somehow 'weak' or 'lacking' in personal resilience. Coleman and Hagell cite research by Ferguson and Horwood (2003) showing that a critical factor in helping young people withstand the impact of major life stressors is access to at least one understanding and supportive adult. When we talk in the following chapters about resilience we mean a capacity to withstand difficulties, setbacks and traumas that is built up and developed within appropriate supportive relationships – be that through family, informal and peer networks or formal service provision – not an innate 'quality' that decides whether you sink or swim. This emphasis on relationships also reflects the views of young people themselves on what they see as central to promoting their health and well-being (Public Health England/AYPH, 2014).

Overall, it can sometimes seem as though adolescence in our society is viewed through a 'pathological' lens – almost as a disease in its own right. This is exemplified by so-called storm and stress models of adolescence, rooted in psychodynamic theories that emphasize the idea of adolescence as a period of crisis. Whilst we would not want to diminish the potential for psychological and behavioural disturbance to arise during adolescence, we would also give emphasis to the fact that the roots of much of this may well lie in the social and cultural context that adults make for them. Maybe, therefore, the way to address many of the health issues that young people face is not to change *them*, but rather to change aspects of the society in which they live. The idea of building resilience in young people should not, we argue, involve helping them to permanently cope with the unfair, the unjust and the intolerable – but to challenge and change the conditions in which they live; resilience should be a platform for empowerment. We would also like to affirm that adolescence is best viewed as a positive life stage, full of hope, wonder and potential, and absolutely to be celebrated!

The structure of the book

The book is structured in two parts. In Part 1 we have three introductory chapters which are intended to lay the groundwork for the issue-specific chapters that follow. After the current chapter, we will move on in Chapter 2 to look at adolescence as a developmental life stage. We outline the physiological, psychological and social changes and transitions experienced by young people, including reference to some relevant theories of adolescence. This reflects our view that a developmental perspective is important in understanding the nature and impact of the health issues faced by young people, and how to respond in ways that are meaningful and effective.

In Chapter 3 we present a brief overview of the history of the health issues and health promotion strategies affecting young people. This chapter is meant to show how the issues have changed as society has changed, and thus to make the important link between young people's health and well-being and the social, economic and political context in which they live.

In Part 2 of the book we go on to discuss a range of specific issues that impact on the health and well-being of young people. First, in Chapter 4, we discuss health, well-being and the environment. Some authors concerned with the health and well-being of children and young people have raised the idea that modern post-industrial societies like the UK constitute an increasingly 'toxic' environment in which to grow up (e.g. Palmer, 2006; Louv, 2010). Factors implicated in this include the increasing physical constriction of the 'outside world' that children and young people access, with much more time spent indoors engaged in 'passive' activities, such as watching TV and playing computer games, and much less time engaged in 'free', unsupervised play and exploration of the world – particularly in 'natural' environments – compared with previous generations. Whilst much of this argument has been polemical in nature, the relationship of contact with the natural environment to the mental and physical health, well-being and development of children and young people has increasingly become the subject of a body of rigorous research (e.g. Barton and Pretty, 2010; Greenfield, 2014; Lewis, 2014). We cast a critical eye over these debates and issues and try to identify some of the important ways in which young people themselves interact with their wider environment.

In Chapter 5, we will go on to look at young people's mental and emotional health and well-being. One of the main concerns currently being expressed about young people is that we appear to be witnessing a marked increase in mental health and emotional problems. To some extent, this continues with some of the themes introduced in the previous chapter; specifically a concern that changes in our society in recent decades are leading to both a 'loss of innocence', as children and young people are forced to 'grow up too quickly', joined with some powerful epidemiological evidence that we are seeing a real rise in mental and emotional health disorders. We consider these debates, and then look at some of the known risk factors, the issues they raise and how they can be responded to, up to and including acute mental health problems. We also look at aspects of the wider social and cultural contexts, and how these relate to the mental and emotional health of young people.

In Chapter 6 we look at the broad area of disability and health in young people. We frame this discussion with reference to five main categories – intellectual disability, neuro-developmental disability, sensory disability, physical disability and long-term or 'chronic' health conditions. Although there is a huge amount of crossover between conditions and categories, we feel it is important to make these distinctions in order to highlight that each of these groups faces distinct, as well as many common, difficulties during adolescence. We go on to look at some of the causes of these conditions, and discuss important changes in the way that disability has come to be conceptualized in recent decades – and particularly the influence of the social model of disability. We then set out a threefold approach to supporting disabled young people which focuses on: 1) the impact of the impairment – stressing the need to understand the way a particular condition impacts on the young person; 2) disabling barriers – looking at and challenging the way the young person is disabled not by their impairment or condition, but by the inadequate or oppressive response to it from society; and 3) a person-centred focus that starts with, and builds upon, a dialogue with the individual young person about what their aspirations are and what support they need to work towards them. We look also at some case studies which outline what this approach might look like in practice.

In Chapter 7 we look at sexual health issues and how they affect young people. Adolescence is often perceived by adults to be primarily about managing the risks associated with emerging sexuality. In many cultures the idea that this is the time when reproduction should begin is not seen as problematic, and it is even encouraged through practices such as arranged marriage. In modern industrial and 'post-industrial' societies such as the UK, however, reproduction in the teenage years has become redefined as a social problem. The reasons for this are complex, relating to concerns about rising numbers of single young mothers and/or young families, who are unable to support themselves financially. The concern often seems to be more about the 'burden' of state welfare support for these young mothers and families than for their health and well-being, although there are legitimate concerns about that and, indeed, the health and well-being of the infants that they raise. These issues are discussed in Chapter 7. So too will a range of other sexual health issues relating to young people, including their vulnerability to abuse and exploitation, and the continued programme to combat the spread of sexually transmitted infections – particularly Chlamydia. This will all be addressed against the backdrop of debates about the so-called sexualization of childhood and the best way to allow young people to attain sexual maturity safely and free from harm and exploitation.

In Chapter 8 we look at nutrition and young people. Recent decades have seen a dramatic change in the nature of our relationship with food in the UK and other similar societies, often driven by powerful corporate and commercial interests. The massive expansion of the fast food industry, the increased use of addictive sugars, salts and unsaturated fats in food production, and the relentless rise of the major supermarket chains have transformed the food environment that children and young people now grow up in. This, together with the rise of an increasingly sedentary lifestyle, has been implicated in the emergence of the worldwide epidemic of obesity, in which the UK is fully embroiled. There is evidence that eating and exercise habits are established early in life for most people, and the rise of obesity in children and young people is a major concern, both in terms of the health and well-being impact on individuals and the management and planning of future health resources. We shall consider debates over how to respond. For example, to what extent should governments regulate the food industry; to what extent should the food industry take responsibility for itself; or should it be parents and/or individual young people who take responsibility for their own eating and exercise habits?

Another area of concern is the rise of eating disorders such as anorexia nervosa and bulimia. Young women in particular seem susceptible to developing these conditions, although increasing numbers of young men are also being diagnosed. Both conditions are usually treated as forms of mental illness and are related strongly to psychological issues of self-esteem and self-perception of body image, both of which undergo significant changes in adolescence. In the modern social context, however, a range of new pressures have emerged, including the influence of computer-manipulated imaging in the fashion industry, and the role of so-called thin sites promoting extreme thinness on the internet. These issues will all be discussed in Chapter 8.

In Chapter 9 we look at substance use and misuse, including illegal drugs, alcohol and tobacco. This is an emotive area of concern, and we focus on an evidence-led approach. We show that concern over the excessive consumption of mind-altering substances is by no means a new phenomenon, and we explore something of the history of this phenomenon. We look then at some of the main substances that cause concern, their effects and impact; and at a variety of theories about why young people take substances, reviewing 'risk' and 'protective' factors, and some of the health promotion responses and treatments used.

Finally, in Chapter 10 we draw some brief conclusions and discuss some of the current and future developments relating to health issues for young people. In particular, we challenge some of the thinking behind the so-called austerity agenda and the current fashion for neoliberal ideology, and argue that an evidence-based 'investment' approach to promoting the health and well-being of young people makes far greater long-term sense, both economically and morally.

Why does it all matter?

This is most succinctly summed up perhaps by medical sociologist and leading researcher in children and young people's health Helen Roberts when she says: 'Investing in child public health is potentially the most important – and most effective – commitment any society can make to its future' (Roberts, 2012, p. 1). In 2011 the UNICEF annual 'State of the World's Children' report chose to focus specifically on adolescence (UNICEF, 2011). The rationale behind doing so was the recognition that the achievements of the UN Millennium Development Programme in improving the health and well-being of children around the world would amount to little if they were not carried through to benefit the world's 1.2 billion young people between the ages of 10 and 19. There was also acknowledgement of the fact that, between the turn of the millennium and the time of writing that report, the global context had changed dramatically in the face of the worst economic crisis since the early twentieth century. The ever-growing and expanding global economy on which so many hopes of development were pinned has gone into contraction, leading governments around the world to impose measures of austerity and to reduce the funds and support available to developing countries from the rich 'developed world'. It also means a new reality of high unemployment and the contraction of opportunities for young people facing the transition from childhood to adulthood – a reality that is being played out in the UK at the time of writing with record numbers of young people classified as 'not in employment, education or training' (NEETs). The impact of the economic crisis on the health and well-being of young people is still really to make itself fully felt, but it is not likely to be anything but negative.

With this in mind we would argue that to focus on the health and well-being of young people is, at this juncture, more important than ever. To back this point, and to conclude this chapter, we reiterate and paraphrase the 'five reasons' to invest in young people given in the 2011 UNICEF report. These are:

1 Because it is right in principle and in line with the UN Conventions on the Rights of the Child.

2 To consolidate the gains made since the turn of the millennium in improving the lot of the world's children. To not see these and other benefits through for adolescents would be both wasteful and demoralizing for young people and their communities.

3 To accelerate the struggle to reduce poverty and inequality. Adolescence is a critical transitional period where cycles of poverty and inequality can either be reinforced or broken. This is as much the case in the UK as elsewhere. Although levels of poverty and inequality may not be as extreme here as elsewhere in the world, they are still important issues to address in relation to health and well-being.

4 Young people constitute the emerging generation who will have to be ready to solve major problems in our society and the world – including unemployment, economic restructuring, environmental crises and overpopulation. They will need all their health and well-being resources to do so.

5 Young people are the future of society, and the world, but they also have a right to live and develop safely in the world in the present. Sadly, they are the section of the population at some of the highest levels of risk of sexual, criminal and economic exploitation, and of being subject to violence and abuse. And not just from 'criminal' gangs or individuals, but also with the more or less direct complicity of governments and corporate interests. They deserve a chance, every bit as much as younger children, to grow up without such threats, and to feel that the society they live in actually cares about them.

One final, but important, point. It is very easy when discussing the health problems and issues facing young people to slip into an overly negative mode. It is important, therefore, to remind ourselves every now and then, as do Hagell, Coleman and Brooks (2013) in their last update of key data on adolescent health, that young people are generally amongst the happiest, healthiest and most optimistic of all age groups in the UK. Most will pass through adolescence and into young adulthood with little or no serious health problems or issues beyond those one would normally expect. In fact, so healthy are young people, for the most part, that the whole emphasis of medicine has been transformed in recent decades. As Hesse and Williams (1995) put it,

> Medicine has changed its focus from acute diseases of children and younger adults to the chronic diseases of the elderly. (p. 122)

It is important to remember, of course, that many of the chronic diseases experienced by older people have their roots in habits and behaviours established in their childhood and youth. We are of the view, however, that young people should be viewed as positive assets to society, and not as some brooding, unhealthy menace, as often seems to be the case in media representations of them – a point made forcefully by the Youth Media Agency in their response to the Leveson Inquiry (2012) into the UK press. Our aim here, then, is to contribute to a positive advocacy for improving and promoting the health and well-being of young people so that as many as possible are able to fulfil the wonderful promise that is the essence of youth.

Suggested Further Reading

Ewles, L. and Simnett, I. (2009) *Promoting Health: A Practical Guide*. London: Bailliere Tindall.

Hagell, A., Coleman, J. and Brooks, F. (2013) *Key Data on Adolescence 2013*. London: Association for Young People's Health.

Hagell, A. and Coleman, J. (2014) *Young People's Health: Update 2014*. London: Association for Young People's Health (AYPH).

UNICEF (2011) *The State of the World's Children 2011: Adolescence: An Age of Opportunity*. New York: UNICEF.

2

ADOLESCENT DEVELOPMENT AND HEALTH

In this chapter we look at adolescence as a life stage, and an important theme will be to explore how we can use that knowledge to promote the health and well-being of young people. Adolescence has been addressed by a wide range of psychological and developmental theorists, and while theories vary, there are some important unifying themes. For example, adolescence is widely recognized as a key period in the development and reshaping of the individual's self-concept and self-image, marked by a profoundly changed sense of identity and self-awareness (Konner, 2010; Kroger, 2004). Whilst a sense of self-consistency is retained, adolescence also marks a significant break with past self-image, social roles and self-evaluation. External sources of evaluation, affirmation and attachment shift markedly away from parents and towards peers generally, and to potential sexual partners in particular. It is also widely agreed that this sense of self is constructed through the restructuring of relationships, via the media of language and behaviour. A positive self-concept is more likely to develop in an individual when the individual's self-evaluation aligns positively with valued and high-status cultural assumptions and ideals.

Although the concept of the 'teenager' may be regarded as a social construct – a cultural product of an affluent industrial/post-industrial society – adolescence itself can be seen as a bio/psycho/social life stage that marks the transition from childhood to adulthood, and particularly sexual maturity. It has been described as a 'critical period' in the human lifespan with regard to health and well-being (Stengard and Appelqvist-Schmidlechner, 2010).

To illustrate this Viner (2012) reminds us that:

- Five of the ten highest risk factors for ill health and disease in adult life – smoking, excessive alcohol use, obesity, low levels of physical exercise and unsafe sex – are most frequently initiated between 10 and 19 years of age.

- This is the life stage where harmful substance abuse is most likely to begin.

- 75 per cent of serious mental health problems are most likely to begin in adolescence, with peak onset between 8 and 15 years of age.

- All-cause mortality rates among adolescents are now higher than for any other life stage apart from newborn infants.

- Morbidity rates due to disability and long-term health conditions, such as type 1 diabetes, begin to rise during adolescence.

Adolescence also presents an important opportunity for health promotion, however, as it is the life stage at which young people begin to 'carve independent lives' and make important health-related choices that can have life-long consequences. Young people also have a high level of 'behavioural flexibility' that offers opportunities for health promotion strategies to influence those choices (Rigby and Hagell, 2014).

The age range of 'young people' as defined by government has varied in recent years, but the recent 'Improving young people's health and well-being' framework document (Public Health England/AYPH, 2014) defines it as age 10 to 24 years. It is important to bear in mind, however, that, although adolescence is often presented as a single life stage there are also stages *within* adolescence. Coleman (2011) makes the important point that there is a considerable difference in the health issues and factors that will be of concern in early adolescence, and those of late adolescence or 'young adulthood'. He advocates the use of a three-stage distinction:

- Early adolescence – typically 11 to 14 years

- Middle adolescence – typically 15 to 18 years

- Late adolescence/young adulthood – typically 19 to 25 years

This is the model we will follow, referring to the different stages within adolescence as they relate to the various issues discussed. This all said, it is still useful to identify key features of adolescence as a general life stage that can inform our understanding of health and well-being, and it is these we will now outline.

Adolescence as a life stage

Adolescence is one of the most dramatic phases of human development and growth, a crucial phase of physiological transition from an immature to a mature adult state – maturity here meaning the capacity to reproduce sexually. In his classic 'stage theory' of lifespan development Eric Erickson (1968) identified adolescence as a critical period of identity formation. He sought to identify the key psychosocial features and 'tasks' associated with each age across the lifespan, and characterized adolescence as a period of 'crisis' for the individual, where childhood identity has to be broken down and rebuilt until maturity is complete and a stable adult identity is attained. Erickson's emphasis on adolescence as a period of crisis has had a strong influence on how this life stage has been subsequently viewed, and echoes of it can be found in much later theory.

Whether the characterization of 'adolescence as crisis' is strictly accurate, the significance of this transition is so important that it is marked in many human cultures by important ceremonies and 'rites of passage' signifying that it is also a cultural transition towards an adult social identity (Konner, 2010). The different facets of the adolescent transition do not necessarily happen in synchrony, however, and there is often a critical gap between physiological maturation and the psychological readiness to cope with the possible consequences.

To make things even more complex and confusing for young people, they are nowadays faced with a barrage of powerful images and messages from various media and marketing sources, as well as moral exhortations from politicians and media commentators, about what being a 'normal' and/or 'successful' young person is. We will explore these cultural messages and their impact later, but we will start by looking at the physiological transitions that mark adolescence.

Physiological development

In biological terms adolescence – particularly early adolescence (11 to 14 years) – represents the final spurt of growth and development into adult physiological maturity. Driven by the genetically programmed release of gonadotropin-releasing hormone (GnRH) targeted at the pituitary gland, a hormonal chain reaction is triggered as luteinizing hormone (LH) and follicle-stimulating hormone (FSH), the so-called pubertal hormones, are released. This happens in both sexes, leading to a rapid phase of growth in height, stature, muscle development and redistribution of body fat; leading in turn to the development of so-called secondary sexual characteristics and, at a biological level at least, the capacity to mate successfully and reproduce (Ford, 2005).

In girls the onset of puberty is usually slightly earlier than in boys, at around the age of 11 to 12 on average in the UK (Hagell et al., 2013). As a rule, teenage girls tend to mature faster and earlier than boys by an average of 2 years or so (Konner, 2010). The hormonal chain reaction centres on the ovaries, leading to an increase in the production of oestrogen, which governs the development of female sexual characteristics. These include the growth of pubic, body and underarm hair, widening of the hips, together with breast and genital enlargement and development. Ultimately, physical reproductive maturation is achieved as ovulation and menstruation become established and regularized. This physiological transformation will usually be complete within 2 years, although, as with almost every aspect of this transition, there is a great deal of variation in the timing and pace of change.

In boys the average age of onset of puberty in the UK is 13 to 14 years (Hagell et al., 2013), and is driven by the release of testosterone from the testes, prompted by the impact of LH and FSH hormones. This initiates a growth spurt, an increase in muscle mass, broadening of the shoulders, deepening of the voice and the development of sexual characteristics. These include growth of pubic, body and underarm hair, genital enlargement and the production of sperm. Although this process is initiated somewhat later in boys than in girls, it tends to last slightly longer, so that boys tend to overtake girls in average height and stature – the so-called sexual dimorphism that is characteristic of human beings in all cultures (Konner, 2010).

The pace and completion of physiological maturation in both sexes does not necessarily tie in with the pace of psychological development – a mismatch which can become a critical factor in some of the psychological difficulties that can be experienced by teenage girls in relation to body image. Simmons and Blyth (1986) developed the 'cultural ideal hypothesis' to describe the relation-ship between the physical changes that occur during adolescence and prevalent sociocultural ideals of appearance and identity, and the way they differ between the genders. In general, the physical changes in boys tend to move them closer to the desired cultural ideal, whilst girls on the other hand tend to move away from the cultural ideal, gaining height, weight and stature. Simmons and Blyth argue that this shift can be particularly significant for early-developing girls and late-developing boys who can experience adolescence as a period of crisis in which their self-image is in conflict with the ideals of appearance and body image to which they are exposed by the barrage of marketing, advertising and popular cultural images directed at them via music videos, TV, film, teen maga-zines and the internet. It is this crisis that appears to be implicated in the devel-opment of eating disorders (discussed in Chapter 8) such as anorexia and bulimia (Papadopoulos, 2014).

Changes in the environment, and particularly diet, can impact on the timing of physiological change in both sexes, and it is this impact that has been impli-cated in the century-long fall in the average age of onset of puberty in Western societies – the so-called secular trend (Konner, 1991). There is also evidence, however, that environmental stress in the form of family disruption, and par-ticularly parental dysfunction, such as substance abuse, domestic violence, paternal absence and criminal offending, can precipitate early onset too, par-ticularly in girls (Tither and Ellis, 2008). Konner (2010) suggests that what might be at work here is an evolutionary strategy noted in a variety of animal species that speeds up physiological maturation in stressful environments in order to allow for earlier reproduction, and thus ensure greater reproductive success, despite the presence of external threats. In modern human societies this may play itself out as a tendency in girls from disrupted family environ-ments to become sexually active earlier, and thus at increased risk of sexual abuse, sexually transmitted diseases and unplanned early pregnancy. Whatever the biological underpinnings, however, there will usually be significant social pressures at work on girls in such situations that will be important in shaping their behaviour. It is important to emphasize always that sexual abuse and exploitation is the fault of the abuser – not the abused. This has, it appears, been all-too-often forgotten by those, including the police and other statutory agencies, meant to be at the front line of protection for vulnerable girls from dysfunctional backgrounds, as the recent spate of abuse scandals in the UK has sadly illustrated (e.g. Jay, 2014).

The physiological transitions in adolescence also involve a range of biochemical changes in both sexes that affect skin, hair and an increased rate of perspiration. Ford (2005) points out that this all requires a new level of self-care and management, heightened further in girls by the demands of managing menstruation. Added to this is the behavioural impact of hormonal changes, including swings in mood and energy levels and an increased need to be restlessly active at some times and for extended periods of sleep at others.

And, of course, there is an increased sexual sensitivity, both in terms of attraction to others, and awareness of, and confidence in, one's own sexuality. Unsurprisingly, this potent mix of physiological and behavioural change requires a significant reorganization of self-awareness and perception that underlies the psychological transformations associated with adolescence. Once again we would emphasize the importance of recognizing that the transitions to physiological and psychological maturity are rarely synchronous. Coleman (1995) has described this as the 'maturity gap', leading often to role confusion, where society expects adult behaviour, but the young person lacks the psychological maturity and experience to deliver it. This can have important implications for mental and emotional health and well-being in some young people as they seek ways to establish themselves in an adult role and identity, perhaps by becoming parents themselves, drinking alcohol and/or smoking tobacco – all social markers of adulthood – but without the resources or experience to manage the full implications of their choices.

Psychological and behavioural development

It has been argued that the whole pace and timing of human development, including adolescence, is centred on the brain (Bainbridge, 2009). The size and complexity of the human brain, plus the complexity of the social and cultural milieu that it has to master and fit in with – the extent of learning it has to undertake – requires an extended period of physiological development, which is essentially what childhood is all about from a biological perspective. Adolescence marks the culmination of that process and is marked by significant brain growth and neurological development, including increased density of brain mass and a reduction in, or 'pruning', of neurological links. This 'pruning' aspect of neurological development might seem somewhat counterintuitive, but can be understood as a process whereby the efficiency of neurological functioning is increased, alongside an increase in the development of processing capacity. It is this process that leads to psychological maturation (Konner, 2010; Seung, 2012).

This manifests itself in some significant ways. For example, there are marked changes in cognitive processing ability, so-called fluid intelligence, including increased speed of information processing; increased use and efficiency of working memory; increased communicative capacity as expressed both verbally and symbolically – for example, in writing and artistic expression – and an increased capacity for abstract thought and reason. This all leads typically to significantly increased academic, intellectual and 'game' performance – in computer-based and puzzle games – as well as sport (Ford, 2005; Konner, 2010).

Emphasizing the importance of 'cognitive maturation', Piaget (1973) famously identified adolescence as the fourth and final stage of a child's intellectual and cognitive development – the stage of 'formal operations', from which emerges the capacity for abstract thought and logical reasoning. During this stage the young person shifts from the relatively simplistic 'concrete' thinking of childhood and becomes better able to understand such things as love, differing 'shades' of opinion, variations in perspective, the construction of logical proof, and moral and ethical values. This period is seen then as marking entry to adulthood not just physiologically and cognitively, but also in the capacity for moral judgement. This is recognized culturally by being given entry into participation in politics by voting; the assumption of adult levels of responsibility for actions and omissions under the law; and the assumption of the capacity to voluntarily choose to engage in sexual activity.

Although this increased cognitive capacity manifests itself equally in both sexes, there are some gender differences. There is evidence, for example, that boys show faster and greater development in 'visual and spatial' acuity, manifesting as an improvement in sporting performance, for example, whereas girls show faster and greater levels of development in 'social intelligence', developing a rather more acute sensitivity than boys to the vagaries and complexities of social relationships (Konner, 2010). It is important to recognize, however, the wide range of variation possible in individuals of either sex. Overall though, as many parents and teachers will recognize, adolescents can become very intellectually sharp, very quickly!

There is also significant behavioural change underpinned by these neurological and cognitive developments. The most obvious of these is an increased interest in, and expression of, sexuality, an interest which is most often heterosexual, but which can also be homosexual (or an interplay of the two). This often involves a major renegotiation of interactions with the opposite sex – or members of the same sex – who are found to be attractive (Bainbridge, 2009). Managing this burgeoning sexuality is difficult for many young people because one of the main sources of support, parents, now become probably the last person they want to talk to about this particular issue. Thus they become reliant on other sources of knowledge – some of which are highly problematic.

The rise in access to, and use of, the internet by young people has led to the concern that many are now using pornography to learn about sexual behaviour. This concern is part of a wider debate about the 'sexualization' of the world young people find themselves in. Recent theorists, such as Ding and Littleton (2005), have focused on the impact of 'consumer culture', arguing that in modern, media-dominated cultures, such as the UK, identity and status are being reconstructed and reshaped through the acquisition and conspicu-ous display of possessions, particularly clothing, fashion and communication technology, such as smart phones and tablets. There is much debate about the impact of information and communication technology on the psychological and cultural environment in which young people find themselves. Although much of this impact is recognized as positive and beneficial, there are con-cerns that its pervasive influence is both adding to and magnifying the pres-sures that adolescents find themselves under at this stage of their lives. In particular, the impact of fashion images, music videos, internet and magazine media, and advertising with its emphasis on highly sexualized images of young women and 'hyper-masculinized' images of young men has been highlighted (Bailey, 2010; Ding and Littleton, 2005; Papadopoulos, 2011). For these rea-sons the need for high-quality sexual health and relationships education (SHRE) in schools, as well as guidance from parents, teachers and other profes-sionals working with young people, has become more important than ever. These are themes and issues to which we will return repeatedly in subsequent chapters.

It is also well established that adolescents, and particularly young men, are more likely to take risks with what can seem little or no fear or acknowledge-ment of the potential consequences – illustrated most tragically by the fact that road traffic accidents are the most common major preventable cause of death among young men in the UK (Hagell et al., 2013). There are a range of theories explaining this. Steinberg (2008), for example, argues that increased risk tak-ing in adolescence is linked to changes in the brain's socioemotional system, which results in an increase in reward-seeking behaviours, especially in the presence of peers. The socioemotional reward system may develop faster in adolescence than cognitive control systems, suggests Steinberg, thus reducing the capacity to inhibit behaviour in risky situations. He goes on to suggest that adolescents are 'hard wired' to take risks as part of growing up and stepping out independently into the world. Similarly, Casey et al. (2008) argue that a lack of impulse control caused by developments in the brain's limbic reward system may be behind increased risk taking, creating a heightened responsiveness to rewards – that is, a 'bigger kick'. They agree with Steinberg's suggestion that for young people some degree of risk taking is inevitable.

These 'biodeterministic' explanations can lead to the rather pessimistic conclusion that no amount of health education is likely to reduce the adolescent tendency to take risks. Others are far more optimistic, however. Rivers et al. (2008) suggest an approach that involves providing detailed information about the health risks to young people, arguing that education should work on what they call the 'gist-based processing system', altering the 'valence', or meaning, of particular risk activities and behaviours. Thus, even if we accept the premise that young people are 'hard wired' to take risks, work on influencing the social meanings of risk-taking behaviours is likely to be more effective than focusing our efforts merely on 'information-giving' interventions.

At the most basic level, education can help young people separate fact from myth. For example, girls may believe that if they have had unprotected sex more than once without becoming pregnant they are likely to be infertile, or that having an abortion makes you infertile. Similarly, young people may have some knowledge about 'units' of alcohol, but underestimate the amount they are drinking, or believe that drinking alcohol is only harmful if you drink so much that you are sick. There is also a more subtle myth among young people: the idea that 'everyone else is doing it', whether that be having sex, drinking alcohol or smoking cannabis. Perceptions of social norms can shape behaviour, and presenting young people with actual statistics about their peer group, as well as helping them think more critically about media messages, can help them take greater responsibility for their own decisions.

It is important also, in areas such as sex and relationships and drug and alcohol education, that the development of interpersonal skills is included, allowing young people the chance to practice assertiveness and negotiation skills. Young people also benefit from time spent exploring their own, and others', attitudes and values, and thinking about real-life situations – for example, the links between alcohol, sex and decision making (Lynch and Blake, 2008). This last point highlights the tremendous value of talking to young people themselves about why they behave in risky ways, and drawing them into evaluating, designing and, ultimately, delivering health promotion strategies. In recognition of this, the development of participatory approaches to health promotion is one of the key recommendations of the Framework for Young People's Health and Wellbeing (2014).

The cognitive and behavioural changes which manifest themselves during adolescence underpin a major shift also in social and cultural relationships, and a fundamental reshaping of identity. This involves a significant renegotiation of relationships with parents, other adults and peers, and also, in Western societies, a transition towards an occupational/career-related identity and economic independence.

Social and cultural development

As observed earlier, many cultures mark the social transition of adolescence with ceremonies and rites of passage, such as the bar mitzvah in Jewish culture, and, more controversially, male and female circumcision, arranged marriage and military service in some cultures (Konner, 2010). In Western cultures the transition to a full adult socioeconomic identity has become increasingly delayed and prolonged, with a greater amount of time spent in education and/or vocational training. This has been reinforced by a popular culture that seems increasingly centred on a perpetuation of adolescence into young (and not so young) adulthood. Adolescence is therefore, at a cultural level, becoming 'stretched' at both the lower and upper age limits. As we have already seen, increasing concern is being expressed that this is leading to the sexualization and commercialization of childhood and adolescence as the music, fashion and other industries look to extend markets for their products by targeting the desire of younger children to look and act older than they actually are (Papadopoulos, 2011; Bailey, 2012). We will return to this issue in a number of subsequent chapters, but there is increasing evidence that it is having a significant impact on the health and well-being of young people in a number of areas, such as increases in eating disorders, and other mental and emotional health problems in recent decades.

Another issue that taxes all known human societies is the management of the propensity for physical aggression in young men (Konner, 2010). This has become a significant problem in societies, including the UK, where increasing numbers of young men, usually in impoverished urban areas, go through adolescence without the restraining control or positive influence of older men, and is further exacerbated when social mobility and economic opportunities, particularly employment, are absent or in short supply. In such environments young men will seek status, material and sexual gratification in whatever ways they judge open to them, often in conflict with the interests of other members of the communities in which they live – and, of course, wider society and authorities. The consequences of this for their own health and well-being, and for others around them, can be devastating, including increased risk of early death, physical injury, substance addiction, psychological trauma and mental ill-health, imprisonment and, consequently, severely damaged life chances; effects that have been powerfully documented across affluent societies by Wilkinson and Picket (2009). This highlights the impact of economic, political and ideological factors on young people's health and well-being – a factor we shall return to consider in later chapters.

One final point to make in concluding this brief overview of adolescence is that the factors that influence development, health and well-being during this life stage do not begin and end there. Each adolescent has, of course, been an infant and a child, and much about how they deal with the transitions of adolescence will have been shaped by what has happened to them in their earlier childhood. Theorists from across the different schools of psychological thought are generally agreed on this, although they may emphasize different aspects of the processes by which it happens. For practitioners working with adolescents and young people this is an especially important point, whatever the context in which they work – health, education, social care or youth work. It may not be necessary, or even desirable, to know all the details of a young person's individual, childhood history, but it is important to remember that they have one, and that what happened to them during their earlier life will influence how they are now dealing with the challenges and transitions of adolescence. Becoming the best resource they can be for the young people they work with will inevitably require practitioners to develop an awareness of, and sensitivity to, this fact.

Implications for health promotion with young people

An understanding of the nature of adolescence as a life stage helps us to recognize that health promotion with young people has particular challenges and features that differentiate it from working with other age groups. This will help ensure that health promotion strategies and activities that engage with young people work in ways that connect with, and are relevant to, them. In particular, we need to remember that:

- Peer relationships replace family relationships in importance during adolescence, so parents and carers can find themselves losing their previously 'omniscient' influence, and certain subjects may become off-limits altogether – sex being perhaps the most obvious!;

- Other 'authoritative' adults – youth workers, teachers, health promotion workers, counsellors and other mentors – may be looked to by young people as sources of neutral and/or judgement-free knowledge, advice and support – particularly around sensitive topics such as sexual health and substance use;

- Young people will increasingly explore many health-related issues for themselves, accessing sources that are hugely variable in terms of quality and accuracy – including peers, the internet and social media. It is important, therefore, that accurate, quality information is as widely disseminated as possible and made easily accessible in places young people are likely to find it;

- We live in an era when young people live with high levels of mental and emotional pressure – from a test- and exam-obsessed education system, intensive and relentless corporate marketing aimed directly at them and often deliberately playing on their insecurities, to a massive expansion in social media and communication technologies which make significant impacts on their time, emotional well-being, sense of identity and self-esteem (Hill, 2014). There are many potential opportunities available for young people in the modern world, but also many pressures that underpin the growing proliferation of mental and emotional health issues in this age group – arguably *the* main health issue of the present day for young people in the UK;

- Poverty and growing social inequality are major risk factors for current and future generations of young people. A significant body of research now exists that shows that societies, such as the UK, which tolerate high and increasing levels of inequality have poorer health and well-being outcomes than those which do not (e.g. Wilkinson and Picket, 2010; Dorling, 2011 and 2014). A major focus of health promotion activity therefore should be aimed at changing society rather than changing young people themselves;

- Above all, we need to promote the idea that adolescence is a life stage, not an anti-social disease! Some sections of the media seem to revel in depicting young people as a threat to social order and civilization as we know it. In reality, young people are more often the victims of crime, exploitation and prejudice rather than the perpetrators – and are currently, as shown by Dorling (2014), one of the social groups most negatively affected by the so-called austerity agenda.

To understand adolescence we need to look at the complex interplay of influences that are both biologically and culturally determined. The physiological transformations that happen during adolescence are determined by a complex interplay of genes and hormones, but environmental factors, such as nutrition, air, water and housing quality, and the stresses and strains of the psychosocial environment also impact significantly. All of the major risk to young people's health and well-being discussed in this book are much more likely to occur where young people also experience poverty, deprivation, poor parental support, disconnection from education and unemployment (Roberts, 2012; Viner, 2012). The health impacts of socioeconomic pressures on young people cannot be underestimated and the impact of these factors will be a recurring theme in the following chapters.

Suggested Further Reading

Bainbridge, D. (2009) *Teenagers: A Natural History.* London: Portobello Books.

Coleman, J. and Hagell, A. (eds) (2007) *Adolescence, Risk and Resilience: Against the Odds.* Chichester: Wiley.

Coleman, J. (2011) *The Nature of Adolescence* (4th edition). London: Routledge.

Viner, R. (2012) Life stage: Adolescence. In *Annual Report of the Chief Medical Officer 2012, Our Children Deserve Better: Prevention Pays.* London: HMSO.

3

HISTORICAL OVERVIEW OF HEALTH PROMOTION AND YOUNG PEOPLE

In this chapter we give a brief overview of the modern history and background of health promotion for young people. The chapter is not intended as a comprehensive outline, but to 'set the scene', as it were, for what follows; and also to highlight the link between social change and young people's health and well-being. The health issues facing young people in the UK have changed significantly over the last century. The main issues that dominated the thinking of those concerned with public health in the late nineteenth and early twentieth centuries included, for example, the control of infectious diseases (such as tuberculosis and polio), the often appalling working conditions (including those of children and young people) in the factories, mines and workshops of the rapidly industrializing towns and cities produced by the industrial revolution – where long hours, low pay and hazardous machinery were the norm – and the equally appalling living conditions in the newly industrialized cities – including air and water pollution, unsanitary and overcrowded housing and poor quality diet (Porter, 1999).

It was from such concerns that the discipline of public health emerged in the nineteenth century, as pioneering doctors, health scientists and social reformers focused on improving public sanitation, air and water quality, sewage disposal, diet, housing conditions and family planning. The Public Health Acts of 1848 and 1875, for example, were primarily concerned with addressing unsanitary and polluted urban living conditions (Porter, 1999). These Acts reflected, in part, concern in the higher levels of the establishment and ruling classes that Great Britain lacked enough fit workers and soldiers with which to extend and defend its massive global economic and military empire, then at the height of its global reach. The political will to generate initiatives to improve the health of school children took hold seriously, for example, when a survey in England just after the Boer War revealed that 70 per cent of young men were 'unfit for war' (Hobsbawm, 2014a).

Public health issues were also a major focus for some sections of the established church (the Salvation Army for instance), non-conformist churches (such as Methodists, Unitarians and Quakers) and the emerging Labour and Trade

Union movements. The latter were particularly involved in campaigns to improve working conditions, and promote the rise of 'municipal socialism' which emphasized improvements in housing, living conditions and infrastructure (Hobsbawm, 2014b).

It was the end of the Second World War in 1945 that proved the major catalyst for a new public health agenda, however, as part of a broad programme of social reform aimed at eradicating what had been described in the influential Beveridge Report (1943) as the 'five great social evils' of the pre-war era:

- Ignorance – via the extension of universal compulsory education

- Want – via a universal social security system

- Idleness – via the pursuit of full employment

- Squalor – via a major house building and urban regeneration programme

- Disease – via the establishment of the National Health Service

The need, literally, to rebuild society from the rubble was seen as an important opportunity also to mobilize the widespread sense of social solidarity generated by the war to rebuild society anew. This idea was encapsulated in the highly successful Labour Party election slogan 'now let's win the peace!', and it was the post-war Labour government that instigated a radical programme of reform aimed at addressing the 'five evils'. At about the same time, the 1944 Education Act – the so-called Butler Act – made it the duty of local education authorities to embrace health as an area of educational concern; a significant policy shift towards using schools as a means to promote the health and well-being of children and young people (Thane, 1996).

The foundation of the National Health Service (NHS) in 1948 created a national, universally accessible health service, free at the point of use, paid for through taxation. Through its various manifestations and reorganizations the NHS has remained the most important agency working to meet the health needs of young people directly in the UK, either in a reactive way by responding to disease, injury and ill health, or in a proactive way via programmes of primary, secondary or tertiary health promotion (such as immunization, vaccination and screening programmes for those at risk of developing health problems), and of targeted care and support for those affected by disease, injury and disabling conditions (Thane, 1996). The NHS is also the main provider of mental health treatment for young people via Child and Adolescent Mental Health services (CAMHs) (discussed in Chapter 8).

The NHS has also undertaken a major health education role in areas such as sexual health and substance misuse, although, since the 1980s, this has been increasingly taken on by private and voluntary sector organizations. The NHS still takes the lead in certain prioritized areas of health promotion, however, such as those currently targeted at cutting the rate of sexually transmitted infections (STIs), and screening programmes for Chlamydia in particular (discussed in Chapter 5).

The rise of 'the teenager'

It has been argued that the phenomena of the 'teenager', as we now understand it, also emerged in the post-Second World War era. For the first time in history, on the back of post-war economic growth, young people began to experience an unprecedented degree of financial affluence, independence and relative freedom. Ogersby (1998) characterized this as the 'explosive' discovery of teenage identity. The 1950s in particular was a decade in which young people as a distinct social group began to carve out a separate collective identity, adopting the hallmarks of fashion and music imported from the main centre of the newly developing consumer capitalism – the USA. Among these 'hallmarks' were cigarettes and alcohol, heavily marketed as symbols of adult glamour, success and style. This era can also be seen, therefore, as marking a significant shift in the health issues faced by young people, away from the infectious diseases and work-related hazards of the pre-war era, and towards the so-called lifestyle-related health issues of the modern era.

In fact, prior to the 1960s little attention was given to the health of young people as a distinct social group. The emergence of such a focus gained impetus with the rapidly changing social and moral climate associated with that decade. The so-called sexual revolution associated with this era was made possible by the new and widespread availability of the contraceptive pill, which gave young women unprecedented levels of freedom, choice and control over their sexual behaviour. At the same time the increasing availability and accessibility of recreational drugs, such as Cannabis, LSD and Cocaine was added to the mix. The late 1960s and early 1970s was the era in which being young came to be inextricably associated with the cultural phenomena of 'sex, drugs and rock n' roll'.

A new generation of health and education professionals, informed by the burgeoning sciences of child development and child psychology, was also emerging at this time. They created new services to meet new challenges, adopting an increasingly proactive model of public health designed to prevent and pre-empt health problems, rather than respond reactively. Traditional programmes, including immunization, vaccination and screening continued, together with established programmes of child health surveillance (measuring and weighing), conducted mainly in schools. But there was an increasing emphasis on health education as part of a newly emerging 'social', as distinct from purely 'medical', approach to health promotion. It was this approach that ultimately came to be embodied in the Ottawa Charter of the World Health Organization (1986), which defined health promotion as:

> ... the process of enabling people to increase control over, and improve their health. To reach a state of complete physical, mental and social wellbeing an individual or group must be able to identify and to realize aspirations and satisfy needs, and to change or cope with the environment. Health is therefore seen as a resource for everyday life, not the objective of living. Health is a positive concept emphasizing social and personal resources, as well as physical capabilities.
>
> (Cited in Ewles and Simnett, 2009, p. 14)

The charter identified five key areas for action:

- *Building Healthy Public Policy*
- *Creating Supportive Environments*
- *Strengthening Community Action*
- *Developing Personal Skill*
- *Reorienting Health Services.*

Importantly, a direct connection was made to political and economic policy making, and an onus was placed on governments to make health promotion an important priority, not just in the provision of health and medical services, but also in wider areas of policy, such as housing, environmental planning and protection, transport and education.

'Lifestyle' health issues, consumerism and technology

The WHO Charter was, in part, a recognition that the new lifestyle-related health issues, such as obesity, heart disease, smoking and diet-related cancers, and type 2 diabetes – the so-called diseases of affluence – were now the main threat to health and well-being in affluent countries. Obesity (discussed in Chapter 8), for example, once a disease of the 'idle rich', has now become much more prevalent in poorer areas in the UK as high-sugar/high-fat diets have been made cheaply and easily available via the boom in fast food culture and supermarket shopping. This, together with greater access to cars, and more sedentary forms of work and leisure, have created what researchers in the United States (where it is even more prevalent) have described as an 'obesogenic environment'; an environment in which it is actually hard *not* to become overweight (Powell, Spears and Rebori, 2010).

Concern over rising levels of obesity has contributed to recent debates about the changing environment in which children and young people are growing up (e.g. Palmer, 2006; Louv, 2010; James, 2007; Dorling, 2011, 2014; Papadopoulos, 2014). These polemics have been linked to a number of reports from high-profile organizations and individuals – some of them government sponsored – highlighting the perceived threats to children and young people's health and well-being from an environment increasingly dominated and shaped by corporate and commercial interests (e.g. Papadopoulos, 2011; Bailey, 2010; The Children's Society, 2012).

It is tempting to think that such concerns are new and novel phenomena, but, in fact, similar debates can be traced back to at least the early post-Second World War period. Young people in the UK and other affluent societies began at that time to have access to unprecedented levels of disposable income, much of which was – and continues to be – spent on the new technologies and status symbols of affluence.

Take transport, for instance. Access to cars, motorbikes and scooters opened up new levels of independence for young people, particularly young men, in the 1950s and 1960s. This, in turn, opened up new areas of risk as the capacity for damage to oneself and others also increased. Risky 'showing off' behaviours in the pre-car era may have occasionally resulted in death or injury, but as access to motorized transport became virtually ubiquitous, they became *the* major cause of death and serious injury for young men – as they remain to this day (Hagell, 2014). When combined with gang cultures, and a propensity for anti-social behaviour, they also became a significant cause of trouble, injury and stress for the communities those young men lived in, or visited, with their new-found mobility. The 'mods' and 'rockers' gang fights in the seaside holiday resorts of the early 1960s can be seen, perhaps, as an early dress rehearsal for much of what was to follow in subsequent decades.

It is easy to overplay the anti-social tendencies of youth cultures, however, creating – as some sections of the press are all too eager to – sensationalized 'moral panics' about the 'degeneration of modern youth' (Muncie, 2010). New technologies gave young people an independence from adult communities and control that allowed them the space to invent their own distinct 'tribal' identities and communities. Most of these 'tribes' and communities were, and continue to be, largely benign, amounting to little more than an attachment to certain forms of fashion and music – which had also become more accessible with the rapid development of audio technologies and electrified musical instruments.

The mass pop cultures that emerged in the 1950s and 1960s were quickly seized upon by a new breed of entrepreneur – Richard Branson for example – who saw the massive market potential of young people as consumers. Since then most affluent societies have witnessed a progressive mass-marketization of youth cultures, punctuated occasionally by bursts of self-generated and self-defined rebellion – such as punk, or hip-hop, for instance. These bursts of rebellion are quickly assimilated, however, by corporate strategists quick to realize that, rather than a threat, they represent new commercial opportunities. These markets were, in turn, fed by new forms of popular media, all plugging into the insatiable adolescent appetite for experimenting with, and reconstructing, identity. Primary among these was television.

It is difficult to underestimate the social, cultural and psychological impact of television, although debate continues to rage about its impact and influence on behaviour – particularly on violence and sexual behaviour. TV has unquestionably reshaped our knowledge, understanding of and interaction with the wider world. Current generations of young people are more informed and aware of what lies beyond their own immediate environment than previous generations. They have also been subject to more advertising, marketing and strategically manufactured cultural influence – high and low – than any generation before them. And most of the subsequent revolution in communication technologies, including smart phones and iPads, represents a development of TV in one form or another. Papadopoulos (2014) has argued that many young people (she focuses particularly on young women) are now living in a primarily visual culture.

Above all, we live now in an 'information age'. The 'traditional media' (TV, radio, newspapers), although all still significant, have been added to by internet and smart phone technology – so-called digital media. The impact of this revolution in media and information technology is now being researched and debated. Some researchers (e.g. Davies, Coleman, Livingstone, 2011; Lewis, 2014), whilst recognizing the dangers and risks – the so-called digital safety issues – are keen to emphasize the positive impacts, particularly in education, entertainment and social networking. Others have raised concerns about deeper impacts on young people's health and well-being. Greenfield (2012), for example, has highlighted the parallel rise in the widespread use of these technologies with mental, emotional and behavioural problems in children and young people. And public concern continues to grow about the exposure of children and young people to pornography, extremist political and religious material (racism, terrorism), sexual exploitation (grooming), online computer gaming and its potential to become addictive and encourage violence, cyber-bullying, and 'unhealthy' influences, such as pro-anorexia and suicide sites. These are all issues touched on in subsequent chapters.

The rise of the new information technologies has been driven primarily by corporate advertising and marketing industries. Advertisers and 'marketeers' know well how easily young (and not so young) people can be made to associate products and brands with the projection of a desirable self-image, their sense of self-esteem, self-evaluation and comparison with others. The fashion, food, drink, music, gaming, information technology and other industries invest heavily in advertising and marketing precisely in order to create and maintain the markets they need to keep increasing their market share and profit growth. As a consequence young people today face a far greater level of marketing media than any previous generation, much of which takes aim directly at the sense of identity and psychological transition which lies at the heart of adolescence. The primary aim of marketing is to generate both desire and discontent; a pervasive sense of having to keep up, a sense of failure if you cannot afford to – and, all too often, arrogance if you can. All of this has an increased impact in societies, such as the UK, which tolerate high, and increasing, levels of inequality.

Reducing health inequalities was a major target of the New Labour governments between 1997 and 2010, and particularly the 2004 Children's Act (HMSO, 2004), which gave legal standing to its 'Every Child Matters' agenda. This agenda set out five main aims for children and young people, to:

1 Stay healthy

2 Be safe

3 Achieve economically

4 Contribute to society

5 Enjoy life

The aim of public services, across the statutory, private and voluntary sectors, was, under this agenda, to help children and young people achieve these aims by working together through multi-agency collaboration, providing extra input and support as and when the need arose.

This agenda was also backed up the Healthy Schools Programme, launched in 1999, the Behaviour and Attendance Strategy (DfES, 2003), and Behaviour and Education Support Teams, all designed to encourage schools to adopt a 'whole-school' approach and integrated support for health and well-being. These initiatives aimed to support children and young people to develop healthy behaviours, reduce health inequalities, promote social inclusion and raise educational achievement levels, focusing on four main areas:

1 Promoting physical health, particularly through the promotion of physical education (PE) and school sports

2 Promoting emotional health and well-being

3 Healthy eating – as part of a broader strategy to counter the rise of childhood obesity

4 Personal, social, health and economic education (PSHE)

Schools were able to attain 'Healthy School' status by working to meet a range of criteria; and a similar approach was also encouraged in colleges and universities.

The 'Every Child Matters' agenda was archived by the Coalition government when it came to power in 2010. Most of the statutory requirements established by the 2004 Act were dropped and replaced by voluntary ones instead. National government funding for the Health Schools programme was also removed. Consequently, the nationwide consistency of the National Healthy Schools System has been replaced by locally driven programmes which vary greatly in quality and commitment from area to area.

These developments are related to wider ongoing debates about the relative roles, responsibilities and relationships between individual young people, their parents and carers, and the State – as represented by agencies and institutions such as schools, the NHS and the welfare benefits system – all set against the background of the so-called austerity agenda, and the government's goal of reducing the budget deficit created in 2008 by the taxpayer bail-out of failing banks.

In terms of health promotion, a significant debate is taking place over the extent to which interventions should be 'targeted' at specific groups – particularly the poorest – or whether they should be 'universal' and aimed at the whole population. The Children's and Families Act (HMSO, 2014), for example, aims to specify the criteria for targeting children and young people with special educational needs (SEN). The stated intention is to clarify for local authorities and parents when it is that a local authority becomes legally obliged to instigate an integrated 'Education, Health and Care (EHC) Plan'. Criteria can be used to exclude as well as to include, however, and many are watching with interest to see the effect this relatively new piece of legislation will have – and particularly if it will result in some children and young people who might previously have received care and support now falling outside the criteria.

Targeting has been critically evaluated in a number of other areas too. Roberts (2012), for example, posed the question in relation to obesity; should we be targeting only the worst – the statistical tail end of the most extreme – or trying to shift the whole population in a healthier direction? The problem with a targeted approach, she argues, is that it can 'normalize' unhealthy behaviours in wider populations, whilst focusing health promotion effort purely on the most extreme cases.

Targeting is sometimes justified on cost grounds, reducing costs by focusing only on the most needy. This may appear to be common sense, but may not, in fact, be the best use of resources, or best value for taxpayers' money in the longer term. For example, cutting funding to youth work projects to save money now could possibly lead to higher future expenditure on dealing with problems related to gangs, violence and anti-social behaviour that arise later. We will return to this debate in subsequent chapters.

The growing impact of inequality

The impact of health inequalities is an increasingly significant debate at the current time. The geographer and social scientist Daniel Dorling (2011), for example, has emphasized the significance of growing inequality in the current era in the UK, where it has now reached levels not seen since the late Victorian era – the time span covered in this chapter. Among the many negative impacts Dorling has highlighted are those related to the physical and psychological health and well-being of children and young people, many of which emerge in the issues addressed in subsequent chapters.

To address health inequalities a growing number of health and social scientists (e.g. Stengard and Appelqvist-Schmidlechner, 2010; Dorling, 2011; Roberts, 2012; Hagell and Coleman, 2014) are asserting that health promotion with young people needs to be seen as an investment rather than a cost burden for society; indeed the 2012 Chief Medical Officers Report (Davies, 2012) was entirely devoted to this argument and the evidence for it. The right type of health promotion enacted now, it is argued, will reduce long-term health expenditure costs for society (e.g. Pretty et al., 2009; The Marmot Review, 2010; Strelitz, 2012). Cutting services to save money in the short term may well incur higher costs later as potential health problems turn into actual crises – the projected future epidemic of type 2 diabetes resulting from high levels of childhood obesity is one of a number of examples highlighted by Strelitz (2012). As Hagell and Coleman (2014) put it:

> ... investing in young people's health provides huge dividends for their current well-being and their future health. Getting it right at this age also reduces long term costs to the health system.
>
> (Hagell and Coleman, 2014, p. 2)

This is an argument we will return to again in our final chapter. But first, let us now look at the various issues that are seen as most significant for young people in the UK today.

Suggested Further Reading

Furlong, A. (2009) *Handbook of Youth and Young Adulthood: New Perspectives and Agendas.* London: Routledge.

Hagell, A. and Coleman, J. (2014) *Young People's Health: Update 2014.* London: Association for Young People's Health (AYPH).

Hagell, A. and Rigby, E. (2014) *The Effectiveness of Prevention and Early Intervention to Promote Health Outcomes for Young People.* Paper prepared for Public Health England Annual Conference, 16/17 September 2014, University of Warwick.

Ogersby, B. (1998) *Youth in Britain since 1945.* London: Routledge.

Porter, D. (1999) *Health, Civilisation and the State: A History of Public Health from Ancient to Modern Times.* London: Routledge.

Roberts, H. (2012) *What Works in Reducing Inequalities in Child Health* (2nd edition). Bristol: Policy Press.

Viner, R. (2013) Life stage: Adolescence. In *Annual Report of the Chief Medical Officer 2013, Our Children Deserve Better: Prevention Pays.* London: HMSO.

4

YOUNG PEOPLE'S HEALTH, WELL-BEING AND THE ENVIRONMENT

The environment is a central health issue in promoting the health and well-being of young people. The Ottawa Charter (WHO, 1986) identified 'creating supportive environments' as one of its five key areas of action for promoting health, highlighting the need to create 'safe, stimulating, satisfying and enjoyable' living and working conditions. The charter advocated that health promotion assessments be built into the design of the environment at various levels, including workplaces, the layout of cities and communities, the impact of energy production and the protection and conservation of the natural environment and resources (WHO, 1986, cited in Hubley and Copeman, 2008).

Ever since the beginning of the industrial revolution there has been concern about the relationship between health, well-being and the environment. As we saw in Chapter 3, the origins of the discipline of public health were rooted in concerns about the physical and 'moral' impact of life in the new, often chaotic and insanitary, urban environments created as industrialists sought to centralize and mechanize the production of goods such as textiles in the eighteenth and nineteenth centuries. The massive wealth that could be generated from industrialization created major incentives to press ahead with urban and industrial development, often without much thought to the consequences for the physical and mental health of the newly created urban populations. Although some enlightened industrialists did address these issues in the design of their factories and the communities around them, most did not, and many of the new industrial towns and cities were heavily polluted, with near-perfect conditions for the propagation and spread of infectious disease (Porter, 2005). Working conditions in factories, mines and workshops were often grim too, involving long fatigue-inducing hours in which a workforce of all ages, from young children to elderly people, were exposed to noisy, dangerous machinery and, often, a cocktail of dangerous chemicals and dust as well.

The unignorable health consequences of this massive environmental transformation created their own political impetus, leading to an often hard-fought revolution in public health. Significant changes in the physical environment resulted, including major improvements in housing, sewage, water and food quality, improved regulation of working conditions and the reduction of wider environmental pollution. Those reforms, together with the development of scientific medicine and the introduction of a comprehensive socialized healthcare system in the NHS, mean that we now live in the UK in a healthier *physical* environment than almost any previous generation. Infectious disease in particular has largely been eradicated as a threat to life for young people, although there are concerns that overuse of antibiotics may lead to this being a temporary rather than permanent state of affairs. And some types of infectious disease, particularly sexually transmitted infections (STIs), stubbornly continue to increase.

The shift to a so-called post-industrial society and a knowledge-based economy in the UK in the early twenty-first century has led to further change to the environment, and a new type of relationship with it, from which a new set of health issues have begun to emerge, many of which affect young people in particular. This has, in turn, prompted debates about the changing environment in which young people are growing up (e.g. Palmer, 2006; Louv, 2010; Greenfield, 2014).

What do we mean by 'the environment'?

The environment can be defined as everything that surrounds us that we are in contact and interact with, but which lies outside of us as discrete, individual beings (Steg, Van Den Berg and De Groot, 2013). This includes the physical and material environment (both the human-made, or 'built', and 'natural' aspects of our surroundings) and the material resources we have access to, such as the basics of food, water, air and shelter. It also includes the 'psychosocial' environment. Human beings are intensely social beings, biologically and psychologically tuned to interact with others from early infancy and on through the lifespan. The social and cultural aspects of our surroundings are hugely important in shaping us both collectively and individually. Given that adolescence is a critical period for identity construction, it follows that we should not underestimate the importance and impact of the social and cultural environment in shaping adolescents' mental and emotional, as well as their physical, health and well-being.

A particularly important factor in shaping the psychosocial and cultural environment in which young people live and develop is the political and economic context. Stott (2000) highlighted factors such as employment, opportunities for social mobility and achievement of 'economic well-being' as having a major and direct impact on health and well-being. And there is now a wealth of epidemiological and other social scientific evidence to show that levels of economic inequality are linked strongly with inequalities in health and well-being outcomes (Wilkinson and Pickett, 2010). Dorling (2011) has charted the rise in anxiety disorders in adolescence in relation to increasing levels of inequality in the UK in recent decades, and the pressures it has placed on children and young people in particular. An ecological view of health and well-being tells us that all of these environmental factors are interconnected, shaping the life chances and opportunities for young people to achieve optimum health and well-being.

What are the issues?

The environmental context affecting young people's health and well-being has changed significantly in recent decades, and despite important improvements in the physical environment, there have arisen a number of significantly detrimental issues in the UK. This was highlighted by the UNICEF/WHO 'Report Card' (2007) which compared the health and well-being of children and young people in affluent societies, and concluded that young people in the UK are the unhappiest in the developed world. The report placed the UK bottom of a league table of 21 economically advanced countries, based on 40 indicators, including poverty, family relationships and health. Among the key findings were:

- A steady rise in child poverty since the 1980s, with 16 per cent of children living in homes earning less than half the national average wage.

- High levels of distrust, with less than half (43 per cent) of children rating their peers as 'kind and helpful'.

- Many families increasingly struggling to find shared time together, with only 66 per cent of families finding time to eat a meal together 'several times' a week.

- A particular problem with alcohol, with 31 per cent of children admitting to being drunk on two or more occasions.

- Increased levels of obesity (10 to 14 per cent) among 2- to 10-year-olds between 1995 and 2004.

- The highest rate of teenage pregnancy in Europe – 40,000 per year under 18.

A follow-up qualitative study conducted on behalf of UNICEF by Ipsos Mori, led by Nairn (2011), sought to delve more deeply into the reasons why the UK had emerged so poorly, comparing the experience of children and young teenagers in the UK with comparable samples from Spain and Sweden, both of which scored significantly better in the 2007 report. This study found that young people in all three countries felt that what mattered most to them were opportunities to go outside, and spend quality time with friends and family. Opportunities to do these things were severely compromised in the UK, however, by time, work and education pressures on parents and children in a strongly competitive, consumerist culture. This report, whose sample was drawn predominantly from the early adolescent age group, highlighted that the negative impacts of inequality, particularly evident in the UK, tended to increase as children entered secondary school, where they began to make comparisons and distinctions between themselves and others using cues linked to the possession of material goods and brands. These findings were echoed also in 'The Good Childhood Report' from The Children's Society (2012), which showed declines across a range of ten indicators linked to the measurement of children's well-being between 8 and 15 years old.

A note of caution is needed in interpreting these findings, perhaps. It could be argued that what is being captured here is a natural increase in anxiety and uncertainty associated with negotiating the demanding transition between primary and secondary education that is quite common in early adolescence. The findings do seem to correlate, however, with a period of notable changes in the nature of childhood, and in the relationship between children, young people and the environment in recent decades. There is evidence, for example, that in developed societies like the UK young people's physical worlds are 'shrinking', and that time spent in virtual worlds is increasingly replacing contact with the outdoor environment. The so-called radius of activity – or the area close to home which children are able to access without adult supervision – has declined by around 90 per cent in recent decades, compared to earlier generations, according to Glaster (1991, cited in Louv, 2010). Sigman (2007) found that many 11- to 15-year-olds spend up to 7.5 hours a day (roughly half their waking lives) in front of either a TV or a computer screen.

Health impacts and 'the changing nature of childhood'

In terms of the impact on young people's health, concerns about physical health have tended to focus mainly on increasing levels of obesity (discussed further in Chapter 8). Recent figures suggest that 31 per cent of young men and 37 per cent of young women are overweight or obese (Hagell et al., 2013). Beyond obesity, Moss (2012) cites evidence of vitamin D deficiency linked to rickets and short-sightedness, significant increases in asthma and a 10 per cent recorded decline in children's cardiovascular fitness in the last decade – all linked to a decrease in the amount of time spent playing outdoors compared with previous generations.

As described in Chapter 5, we are also witnessing rising rates of mental and emotional health problems, and neuro-developmental disorders such as Asperger's syndrome, Tourette's syndrome and Attention Deficit Hyperactivity Disorder. Moss (2012) cites evidence that up to one in ten children between 5 and 16 years of age are currently diagnosed with a mental health problem; one in twelve adolescents have engaged in self-harm, and around 35,000 children have been prescribed anti-depressants in England. Citing child psychologist Tanya Byron, he argues that the shift away from outdoor play is leading to a decline in opportunities for children and young people to develop important resilience-building skills, such as the ability to assess and cope with risks and challenges.

Much of the debate about these issues has been driven by the work of journalist Richard Louv in the US (2010), and educationalist Sue Palmer in the UK (2006). Louv originally published his bestselling book *Last Child in the Woods* in 2010, and although it focused primarily on the US, it has also become influential in the UK. Its main thesis is that we are currently raising a generation of children and young people experiencing what he calls 'nature-deficit disorder'. Increasing numbers of young people are growing up without having the level of access to 'natural' environments that previous generations did, or the opportunities for 'free' – as in unmanaged by adults – and creative play. Louv recognizes that his view might be perceived as mere nostalgia, so he musters a range of psychological, health and educational evidence for the importance of 'natural play' for physical, psychological and social development and well-being. He argues strongly for a number of responses at parental/carer level – but also at wider political, economic and institutional levels. In particular, he argues for the need to get young people outdoors and into contact with the natural world – and to plan cities, communities, schools, institutional and work environments to build in access to green space.

In the UK, the educationalist and writer Sue Palmer, in her best-selling book *Toxic Childhood* (2006), made a similar argument, focusing on changes in lifestyle in recent decades that have impacted on childhood and parenting. The main issue for Palmer is the changing nature of children's play and its increasing dominance by screen-based technologies since the 1990s. She relates this shift to the progressive commercialization of childhood that has occurred since the 1950s, and a calculated corporate agenda to turn play and entertainment into something to buy, rather than something children and young people create for themselves in interaction with the world and others around them. The corporate role in this process has been made increasingly explicit in what Palmer describes as 'an explosion' of marketing aimed directly at children and young people. She cites, for example, the 'playground culture' peer pressure/pester power chain of effect designed ultimately to pressurize parents into buying whatever the latest 'must have' possession is. Palmer has also mustered a body of research evidence to back up her thesis, and has also paid particular attention to the impact of poverty, highlighting the fact that children and young people from poorer families are particularly vulnerable to the most negative impacts of these trends. Palmer has been criticized by some for being alarmist and 'melo-dramatic' (e.g. Bragg, Kehily and Montgomery, 2013), but her argument does seem to chime with an increasing body of research evidence.

An influential scientific contribution has come from Jules Pretty and his col-leagues at the University of Essex. Rather than focus on negative factors their approach has been to research the positive effects of 'green exercise' – that is, exercise, play and activity in natural environments. They have identified an array of positive physical and mental health benefits, including weight loss, improved cardio vascular fitness, improved mood, self-esteem, stress and anxi-ety levels (Pretty, Peacock and Sellens, 2005). Much of this research has focused on the benefits for the population in general, and for people with mental health problems in particular. In a 2009 report, however, Pretty et al. (2009) emphasized the significant benefits of getting children onto a 'healthy life-path' involving green exercise. This, and a growing body of other evidence (see, for example, Van den Berg, Joyce and de Vries, 2013), leaves little doubt that what most of us feel intuitively – that getting children and young people outdoors and active is good for them, physically, mentally and socially – is actually true.

Young people engage with the physical environment in a wide variety of ways, but perhaps one of the marked features of the modern social context is the extent to which this engagement is orchestrated and organized by adults. To some extent, this has always been the case, and many youth organizations, such as the Scouts, Guides and The Woodcraft Folk, have a long history and tradition of getting young people out in the natural environment for the benefit of their health, well-being and development. More recently, they have been joined by conservation organizations, such as the Wildlife Trusts, The National Trust, the Royal Society for the Protection of Birds (RSPB), The Woodland Trust and others who have actively promoted the involvement of children and young people via dedicated children's and young people's sections, and who have recently sought to combine their efforts through the 'Wild Network'. All of these organizations report a falling off of membership and involvement as children hit the teenage years, however.

Palmer argues that the pressure for young people to disengage with the outside world has become more concentrated in recent years with the rise of child- and teenage-specific TV channels, and the spread of 'smart phone' tech-nology that allows young people direct, and largely unsupervised, access to the internet. This, combined with increased parental paranoia about the 'dangers of the outside' has led to young people spending increased amounts of time indoors, and indeed, in their own room. Echoing earlier work by American child psychiatrist Susan Linn (2004), Palmer pulls no punches in describing this process as nothing less than the 'stealing of childhood'; a hostile hijacking designed to redefine children and young people as consumers, and break childhood down into 'units of consumption' (Palmer, 2012).

It has also been argued that the changing environment of childhood and adolescence is acting not just at a social and cultural, but at a neurological level – literally changing the pattern of brain development, and, ultimately, the very nature of the mind itself. For example, Jackson (in Newnes and Radcliffe, 2005) cites research that suggests that technologies such as television, video games and the internet are changing brain development in affecting the way in which children relate to their environment and other people. Similarly, DeGrandpre (2000) argues that we have developed what he calls a 'rapid fire culture', leading to a constant pursuit of stimulation and a reduced ability to concentrate and/or attend to mundane activities – all symptoms of Attention Deficit Hyperactivity Disorder (ADHD).

The neurological case has been put most comprehensively, however, by neuroscientist Susan Greenfield (2014), who argues that we are witnessing a major qualitative change in the environment in which children's and young people's brains and minds are developing. She describes this as 'mind change', likening the potential impact on society to that of climate change. The rising use of social networking sites is, she argues, eroding social competence as the rich social, physical and sensory realities of real-life communication are replaced with impoverished screen-based versions. Referring to the work of Carr (2010) and Turkle (2010), Greenfield argues that this is contributing to an erosion of empathy and trust among young people, exemplified by a rise in 'online' and 'offline' bullying, as well as a decline in opportunities to learn the subtleties and richness of communication, such as the use of metaphor, associative meaning and abstract thought. She echoes DeGrandre's point – arguing that the rise in computer gaming can be linked to the rise, over the same historical period, in the incidence of ADHD. Computer games offer, she suggests, a more stimulating, exciting, instantaneously rewarding and 'sensational' environment than the 'real world'. Constant or frequent use is associated with the release of dopamine in the brain, the neuro-chemical basis of addictive behaviours. Dopamine inhibits activity in the pre-frontal cortex, an area of the brain associated with higher level cognitive activity, including the generation of 'meaningful' associations. An impact of increased dopamine levels is to increase the need for ever higher levels of sensation and reward-seeking behaviour, where 'sensation trumps cognition' and 'thrills trump consequences' – and many of the behaviours we have come to associate with ADHD, including reduced attention span, low levels of concentration and increased recklessness. The violent nature of many of these games can also, she argues, be linked to an increase of 'low-grade' hostility, particularly among boys and young men. She also suggests a link to other addictive behaviours, including to food, for example, and thus to obesity (Greenfield, 2014).

These are controversial arguments, and the research base for them is rather tentative at the present time. Indeed, there is a counter-body of evidence highlighting the benefits of computer gaming in developing aspects of cognitive performance (e.g. Dye, Green and Baveleir, 2009), and recent research on internet use by children and young people highlights the many benefits that it brings, alongside the risks (e.g. Livingstone, Haddon, Gorzig and Olafsson, 2011; Hill, 2014). The debate on how children and young people engage with technology and the environment is well and truly underway, however, and a great deal more research will undoubtedly follow.

Health, well-being and the environment

In terms of what we know about the relationship between health, well-being and the environment, Konner (1982) has argued that this is shaped by our evolutionary heritage. As a species, *Homo sapiens* evolved to be physically active in an environment that is biologically rich, although with a high degree of unpredictability, in the seasonal availability of food – a reality reflected in the lives of many hunter-gatherer societies to this day. Modern lifestyles, in which we have continuous access to plenty, and increased levels of physical inactivity, are compromising this, however. For instance, because of the unpredictability of food supplies during much of human evolution we have, as a species, been under almost constant selective pressure to develop a physiology that is highly efficient at laying down fat *and* adjusting our metabolism to burn less energy during periods of restricted food intake. The result is the human tendency to put on weight easily, and to find it harder to lose weight when we diet (Diamond, 2012). Herein lie the biological roots of our modern day obesity problem, exacerbated by what has been described by US researchers as an 'obesogenic environment' – a social environment which maximizes passive and sedentary forms of work and leisure, and at the same time actively promotes easy access to a high-fat, high-sugar diet (Powell, Spears and Rebori, 2010).

As well as physical health, clear links are known to exist between levels of physical activity and mental health. Psychologically, we know that access to green views and green space are good for mental health and are 'psychologically healing' (Barton and Pretty, 2010). Cognitively, rich and varied natural environments are also known to be rich learning environments – natural laboratories for learning maths, science, literacy and social skills, and developing resilience to physical and psychological injury and setbacks. Socially, participation in the sort of physical activities that occur in natural play settings involves elements of risk self-management, mental and physical challenge and cooperative planning and action. There is now a strong body of evidence to suggest that all of this is particularly beneficial, both therapeutically and educationally, for children and young people (Maudsley, 2007).

Outdoor and adventure education is being increasingly recognized as a way of working therapeutically with some groups of troubled young people. For example:

'Getaway Girls' – a project based in Leeds which runs programmes and activities aimed at young women who have experienced problems and discrimination associated with structural inequalities, such as poor housing, education and employment opportunities, and who often demonstrate self-harming, violent and challenging behaviours. The project helps them to develop confidence and self-esteem, and to understand and work cooperatively with others through pro-social group learning activities in the natural environment (Carnea, 2008).

'Mentro Allan' – based in Wales, this project targets hard-to-reach groups, including troubled and disabled young people, using outdoor and adventure activities to help them improve health, well-being and confidence (Mattingley and Harry, 2008).

'Get Hooked on Fishing' – based in Durham, the 'Get Hooked on Fishing' project works with troubled young men, using fishing as an activity to divert them away from crime, substance abuse and anti-social behaviour, and to help them develop skills and self-confidence, including the development of a peer-led coaching scheme, where some of the young men go on to teach and coach others (Watson, 2008).

Sport and other strategies

Sport is undoubtedly the main medium through which most young people are encouraged to engage in physical activity, often, but not exclusively, in outdoor environments. As Coleman (2010) points out, there is a wide consensus that engagement in sport and exercise is beneficial for young people. The opportunity to develop and demonstrate physical skills and abilities, enhance physical fitness and stamina, perform and succeed competitively and receive adult and peer recognition for doing so are all likely to have positive psychological, as well as physiological, impacts. Self-esteem and self-confidence are likely to be enhanced, and the known biochemical enhancement of mood and well-being that comes with exercise is also likely to act as a powerful motivator.

Sport can also be a great social leveller, offering young people from impoverished and deprived backgrounds an all too rare opportunity to compete on an even footing with those from wealthier and more privileged backgrounds. The potential material and social status rewards of succeeding at a professional level in some sports – football being the obvious example – offer a particularly enticing pathway for young people who may otherwise find few other ways to achieve personal success and upward social mobility. This all adds up to a very powerful set of motivators.

Teenagers and young adults are also among the most avid and frequent participants in 'adventure' and 'life-style' sports, ranging from skateboarding, surfing and snowboarding, to more 'extreme sports' such as base jumping and bungee jumping. Some of these activities are more accessible to young people from wealthier backgrounds, due to the costs of travel, equipment and tuition. Some, however, as illustrated in the cult film 'Dogtown and Z Boys', start off as part of youth counter-cultures in deprived urban environments, and involve an overt rejection and consciously anarchistic challenge to adult organization and control. Skateboarding and BMX biking, for instance, often involve a deliberate move away from adult-created skate parks, engaging with the wider built and urban environment as an obstacle course – with one aim being to stay one step ahead of the adult authorities who keep that environment under surveillance. These counter-cultural activities have generated their own fashion, music and art, some of which has, inevitably, been usurped by corporate interests and turned into lifestyle brands.

Engagement in sport and outdoor activities can be problematic for some young people, however. Adolescence can be a time of intense self-consciousness and physical embarrassment, and being forced to expose all, or parts, of your body and participate in physical activities that you find difficult, or in which you have no intrinsic interest, can lead to acute physical and psychological discomfort that can have exactly the opposite effects described above. This is particularly true for young people with neuro-developmental conditions such as Dyspraxia, Autistic Spectrum Conditions or Tourette's syndrome (Hendricx, 2010). These are important factors for adults organizing activities to recognize. It may be unfashionable to say it – but sport is not necessarily for all.

Recent governments, concerned about the rise and potential future cost of obesity in particular, have promoted a variety of strategies focusing strongly on exercise and diet, aimed primarily at children and young people – such as the 'The Change for Life' programme. Another example is the well-respected and long established Forest School movement, which originated in Sweden in the 1950s. Despite the strong educational and health-related evidence base that underpins the Forest School approach, it remains largely the province of the voluntary sector in the UK, rather than being incorporated into the state education sector (Lovell and Roe, 2009). Also, the Forest School movement has tended to focus mainly on school-age children, with young people in early adolescence at the top end of the age range.

We have already noted that the UK has a long-established tradition of outdoor educational and youth work organizations, including the Scouts

(Explorers), Guides, Woodcraft Folk and Duke of Edinburgh Awards scheme. These, and the growing conservation and environmental movements, have also pioneered children's and youth groups such as the Wildlife Trusts' 'Wildlife Watch', and The Royal Society for the Protection of Birds' 'Wildlife Explorers'. These movements and initiatives are very much 'owned' and driven by adults, however, concerned both with the healthy development of young people and the conservation of the natural world. It is also recognized that the most successful initiatives in engaging with children and young people are those that connect with intrinsic motivators. Most children are naturally fascinated by animals, 'creepy-crawlies' and the natural world. The continuing popularity of zoos (still the world's most popular day out) and the Natural History Museum in London, for example, are evidence of that. But what about teenagers? Why does it – and does it actually – suddenly become 'uncool' to continue this interest in their early teens? Which strategies might be best aimed at young people to keep them engaged, or to engage them for the first time, with the natural world or 'the outdoors', with all the health and well-being benefits that accrue?

Perhaps the key factors are to ensure, first, that young people can actually access green spaces and places, and second, that a link is established between the activities they can participate in and what matters to them most at this life stage – including how they appear to others (especially their peers), and how what they do relates to their growing sense of their own identity.

Access will obviously depend on the resources and amenities available. The Ottawa Charter, cited at the beginning of this chapter, argued that young people's access to green and open space is as important as access to clean water and healthy food (WHO 1986). Access often depends, however, on the attitude of adults. Young people gathering in parks and open spaces are often viewed with suspicion or hostility by adults who see them as a potential threat to peace and social order. Changing such perceptions is an important part of the need to build trust between older and younger people

Another factor is how such activities relate to young people's often acute concern with how they appear to others – particularly their peers. In the 'Getaway Girls' project, for example, Carnea (2008) notes that body image and appearance is often a central concern of the girls who participate, and that getting the girls to wear the appropriate clothing and equipment is a major task in itself. In outdoor and adventure activities therefore, as in many areas of sport, thought needs to be given to issues of appearance, image and gender mix.

In truth, a lot of young people need no encouragement to engage creatively and actively with their environment – natural or urban! Despite worries over their health and well-being, it is worth bearing in mind, for example, that obesity levels are actually at their lowest among the 16- to 20-year-old age group.

Young people, particularly young adults, are also often the most active in environmental and conservation groups. Conservation and environmental projects are also one of the most common choices for gap year projects among teenagers between leaving college and going to university, and among volunteer projects for university students. All of these are strong indicators that many young people – perhaps more than some concerned adults believe – are actively engaged with following a healthy life path.

Risk factors

Many young people like to push boundaries and take risks (as discussed in Chapter 2). It is sobering to remind ourselves that the top three causes of death in young people generally, and young men in particular, are road traffic accidents, fires and drowning (Patton et al., 2012). Not all of this is due to the recklessness of young people, however. Roberts (2012) reminds us of the important fact that there is a direct relationship between the likelihood of a young person dying or being seriously injured as a result of an accident and their socioeconomic background. Poorer young people tend to live in more hazardous environments. For example, a child or young person from the lowest income groups in society is around six times more likely to die in a house fire. The reasons for this include poorer quality housing and electrical appliances, lower usage of smoke alarms and a higher likelihood that adults and young people in the household are smokers. From 0 to age 5, most fatal or serious accidents occur in the home, but from age 5 up to young adolescence road traffic accidents take over as the main cause. Roberts' review shows that it is actually adults who are culpable for this situation, either as the drivers in most cases, or as the designers and planners of unsafe environments. She also points out that this is an area where well tried and tested environmental adjustments – such as lower speed limits and traffic calming measures – are relatively simple to implement. The political will to override the objections of the motoring lobby seems to be one of the most important factors in doing so. It is questionable whether politicians, or the wider public, would tolerate such a high rate of death and serious injury to young people caused by anything else. Hagell et al. (2013) point out that death or injury caused by violence tends to draw far more attention from the media, for example, despite the fact that it is considerably rarer. The World Health Organization has recognized this issue, organizing large scale global campaigns such as the 'Safe Communities Programme', aimed specifically at reducing the number of injuries and deaths caused on the roads, in young men in particular. There are also signs that the issue is moving up the political agenda in the UK. The Coalition government in the UK initiated moves to make the driving test tougher, and to introduce a probationary period for new drivers. It will be interesting to see if these measures have an impact on the disturbing statistics.

Road traffic accidents are not the only risk, of course. The extreme sports cited above are extreme precisely because of the element of risk involved; and many of the other examples cited, such as skateboarding, BMX biking, surfing and snowboarding, carry a raised risk of injury, if not death. Indeed, part of the 'folklore' of the subcultures that build up around these activities is often based on tales and stories of broken limbs and 'close shaves'. Few would argue that we should ignore such risks and not try to minimize them. Part of the induction into many extreme and adventure sports and activities is highly organized, and involves careful training in the use of appropriate equipment and risk-reducing procedures – the 'buddy' system in scuba diving, where people are trained to dive only in pairs, and to check and monitor each other's, as well as their own, equipment and safety, is an example. And in many 'extreme' activities, such as parachuting or bungee jumping, the organizers themselves take charge of the safety aspects, are legally required and licensed to do so and have a very good safety record as a result.

The fact is, however, that the risk and resultant thrill is often part of the fun for young people. Managing, assessing and responding to risk can also be seen to have a positive intrinsic value for the development and education of young people. For most risky sports and activities there is no doubt that this does need to be overseen by trained and responsible adults. Ultimately, however, it is very unlikely that any society will be able to persuade its young people to risk assess everything they do – and that maybe education and advice may be all that adults can do in many cases.

Conclusions – engagement on their own terms

Underpinning many of the activities and examples described above is the obvious fact that adults will be in charge, at least at the organizational level. At one level, this is no more than a reflection of the reality that much sporting and outdoor activity is organized through schools, or under the auspices of youth or conservation organizations – and sometimes, as we have seen, as a targeted response to the needs of troubled and vulnerable young people. To some extent, however, it also reflects an underlying idea that 'left to themselves' young people cannot engage with the environment in healthy ways. This is a controversial view, however. Many young people engage in sports and games, like football, basketball, volleyball and frisbee, spontaneously – although it is perhaps more likely to be boys than girls that do so.

If we look at what young people actually gain in terms of physical and mental health benefits from such activities, however, then it may not be that different from what is gained from participation in more conventional, adult supervised sports – and some benefits perhaps, such as learning to assess and manage risk, and deal with and become resilient to physically and psychologically painful failure, may actually be greater in some cases. In some activities – notably, surfing – there are also strong elements of community and a powerful, even spiritual, sense of engagement with the natural world. Surf culture also has a strong tradition of environmental activism, exemplified by the 'Surfers Against Sewage' organization.

All of this suggests perhaps that we need to take a rather more nuanced, and young person-centred, perspective on young people's interaction with the environment. Just because their interaction doesn't look like something adults would identify as 'quality', or constructive activity or interaction with the environment, doesn't mean that it isn't so in the eyes of young people themselves. Each generation has to discover its own relationship with the environment it finds itself in, and older generations are perhaps bound to worry about how the next generation will go about doing this. In affluent societies like the UK, the relationship that generations growing up in the post-Second World War era had with the environment was, as in so many other aspects of life, highly unusual. The late twentieth century saw a level of affluence, leisure time and freedom of movement that allowed a whole new relationship with the environment to emerge – one based on appreciation of its beauty, therapeutic, aesthetic and, even, spiritual value.

We are moving now into a new situation. We are now seeing generations of parents who have themselves often grown up without much contact with, or direct experience of, the natural world. For some, like Susan Greenfield, Sue Palmer and Richard Louv, the omens as they stand are grim, and they argue that negative change is being played out in the reality of increases in mental, emotional and behavioural problems, obesity and declines in empathy and resilience in young people. Others have argued that they are being overly alarmist. It is certainly the case, however, that one of the most effective and economically sound ways of promoting the health and well-being of young people, and indeed whole populations, is to promote easy and regular access to a healthy, 'green' environment. That has long been recognized by those working to promote the health and well-being of young people, and, in that respect at least, nothing has actually changed.

Suggested Further Reading

Barton, J. and Pretty, J. (2010) What is the best dose of nature and green exercise for mental health? A meta-study analysis. *Environmental Science & Technology.* doi: 10.1021/es903183r.

Louv, R. (2010) *Last Child in the Woods: Saving Our Children from Nature-Deficit Disorder.* London: Atlantic Books.

Pretty, J., Angus, C., Bain, M., Barton, J., Gladwell, V., Hine, R., Pilgrim, S., Sandercock, G. and Sellens, M. (2009) *Nature, Childhood, Health and Life Pathways.* Interdisciplinary Centre for Environment and Society (iCES) Occasional Paper 2009-2. Colchester: University of Essex.

Van den Berg, A., Joyce, Y. and de Vries, S. (2013) Health benefits of nature. In Steg, L. et al. (eds) *Environmental Psychology: An Introduction.* Oxford: Blackwell/British Psychological Society Textbooks, pp. 47–56.

5

MENTAL AND EMOTIONAL HEALTH AND WELL-BEING

In this chapter we focus on the emotional and mental health of young people. There is widespread concern about this issue, and we appear in the UK to be experiencing an upsurge in mental and emotional health problems in children and young people (Hagell, 2012). For example:

- Up to one in ten children and young people currently experience diagnosable mental health problems, including anxiety disorders, obsessive compulsive disorder and depression, with Hagell et al. (2013) stating that '..... around 13% of boys and 10% of girls aged 11-15 have mental health problems' (p. 77).

- Up to one in twelve adolescents are engaged in some form of self-harm (Moran et al., 2012).

- Conditions such as anorexia, bulimia and eating disorders – all regarded as mental health disorders – now account for the largest number of hospital admissions for 15-year-old girls (Hagell et al., 2013).

- Up to 75 per cent of serious mental illnesses have their onset in early adolescence (Viner, 2012).

Concern is not limited to the UK. A World Health Organization report in 2001 estimated that up to 20 per cent of young people worldwide are affected by a disabling mental health condition, although this is almost certainly an underestimate. Evidence from around the world suggests that young people generally, and young men in particular, are unlikely to look for help and support in dealing with mental health problems, and that those most in need are often the least likely to seek help (Biddle et al., 2004; Rickwood et al., 2005; Sourander et al., 2004; Tylee and Walters, 2004). A particularly alarming statistic is the rise in the incidence of suicide in young men, which by 2001 had become one of the top three causes of death in many European countries (WHO, 2001). More recent research suggests that the suicide rate for young men in the UK has actually fallen somewhat since then, to 13.3 per 100,000 in 2011 (Hagell et al., 2013).

There is no room for complacency, however, and there are fears that the record rates of unemployment among young people that we are now witnessing across Europe, averaging around 21 per cent across the European Union, may begin to push the figure up again.

Stengard and Appelqvist-Schmidlechner (2010) characterize this situation as the 'new-morbidity' of mental health, behavioural and educational difficulties among young people that has become a particular feature of affluent societies since the mid-twentieth century, displacing pre-existing morbidity associated with infectious disease, and leading the WHO to identify mental and emotional health problems as a major area of concern for professionals and policy makers. They highlight the particular vulnerability of young people to social exclusion if they fail to connect with pathways into education and work, leading to a sense of failure and disconnection which can have a highly negative impact on their self-confidence, self-esteem and identity, and a potentially devastating impact on their future. This can include problems associated with poverty, stress, substance misuse, exploitation and involvement in, or becoming the victim of crime. Other knock-on effects include negative impacts on families, friends and wider communities, and major cost burdens for health, social care and penal systems.

We will begin by outlining some of the recent debates around this issue, making particular reference to the concept of resilience. In our discussion we will adhere to the assertion by Weare (2005) that a holistic and preventative approach to mental and emotional health and well-being is the most useful one at all levels, from individual to societal. This builds on the approach identified in the World Health Organization's 'Ottowa Charter' (WHO, 1986), which argued for a focus on the enhancement of positive health characteristics and resources – an approach echoed in relation to mental and emotional health by Stengard and Appelqvist-Schmidlechner (2010). This approach places a strong emphasis on understanding the social and cultural context in which young people live, and the pressures to which they are subject. Such an approach points the way to strategies, from the design and delivery of mental health services for those who need them; to wider networks and systems of support in local communities; institutional support – especially in schools; and the broader political and economic context which underpins it all. If we are going to create a society that is more competent in promoting and responding to mental and emotional health and well-being in young people, then it is important to address all of these strategies.

Mental and emotional health and well-being

According to the NHS Health Advisory Review on Child and Adolescent Mental Health Services (1995), the main components of mental health in children and young people are:

- The ability to develop psychologically, emotionally, intellectually and spiritually

- The ability to initiate, develop and sustain mutually satisfying relationships

- The ability to become aware of others and to empathize with them

- The ability to use psychological distress as a developmental process so that it does not hinder or impair further development

More recently, the 'Young Minds' charity (2014) summarized emotional and mental health as, 'happiness, integrity, creativity; and the capacity to cope with stress and difficulty', relating it strongly to the concept of 'resilience'. The concept of resilience has become increasingly important in discussions around these issues in recent years, with concerns that current generations of children and young people are showing declines in their capacity to deal with life's inevitable difficulties and obstacles.

Resilience has been defined by Newman (2004, p. 3) as 'positive adaptations in the face of severe adversities'. He argues, with reference to the seminal work of Rutter (1987), that resilience is usually seen as a positive quality that relates to both the capacity to deal with stress and the capacity to maintain hope and optimism despite difficulties that may be encountered. It has been described from a social-ecological perspective as, '... both individual processes that increase survival and protective processes instigated by larger systems to provide opportunities for individuals to cope under stress' (Ungar et al., 2013). It is also intertwined with the concepts of 'vulnerability', 'risk' and 'protective factors'. Discussion around the interplay of these factors has grown and, more recently, a preoccupation with 'risk' has begun to give way to a greater emphasis on understanding factors that promote resilience.

Research into resilience in young people strongly suggests that it is often related to their previous experience as children and infants. Of particular importance is the impact of family life and the extent to which the young person has experienced a nurturing and emotionally supportive early and middle childhood – known to be an important protective factor. There is increasing evidence that the foundations of mental and emotional health are actually laid down during early infancy, with deprivation of quality interaction with care givers, and a failure to develop a secure attachment with at least one adult at that stage, strongly implicated in poor mental and emotional health outcomes in later life – with knock-on effects stretching over the entire lifespan (Leach, 2010).

The influence of infant experience on later emotional and mental health is one of a number of risk factors that have been identified relating to significant changes in the nature of childhood in affluent societies in recent decades. This is a central theme of authors such as Linn (2004), James (2005), Louv (2005) and Palmer (2006), who draw on an increasing body of research evidence to support their argument that changes in the nature of children's play, education, use of digital technologies, together with aggressive targeting by corporate marketing strategies, are all playing a part. As we saw in Chapter 4, the neuroscientist Susan Greenfield (2014) has argued that this constitutes a major qualitative change in the environment in which children's and young people's brains and minds are developing in the modern world, arguing that it is literally 'changing brains'. She goes so far as to liken the potential impact on society to that of climate change, raising particular concerns about the impact of significant increases in the time children and young people spend on screen-based activities – a phenomenon described by Jackson (2005) as the creation of 'cybernetic children' – on their capacity to develop empathy and the rich communication skills needed to develop and maintain interpersonal relationships; both recognized as important in the development of strong mental and emotional health.

This argument is given greater force by research such as that conducted by Romano, Osborne and Reed (2013), who found 'withdrawal-like symptoms' in young people making heavy use of the internet when they come offline. They also noted negative impacts on mood and wider mental health, including symptoms of depression, 'impulsive nonconformity' and 'autism-like traits'. And recent neurological studies focusing on adolescents and young adults experiencing 'internet addiction' undertaken in South Korea and China have also tended to back Greenfield's hypothesis (e.g. Hong et al., 2013; Yuan et al., 2011).

There remains controversy surrounding the views of Greenfield and the other authors cited above. They are, after all, challenging some very powerful vested interests. They have, nonetheless, played an important role in initiating a debate, and encouraging a research agenda, exploring the relationship of these factors to what is now widely recognized as a decline in children's and young people's psychosocial health. We will return to look at broader social and cultural factors influencing young people's mental and emotional health at the end of this chapter, but we will now focus on discussing known risk factors.

Known risk factors

Bailey and Shooter (2009) have identified the main known risk factors impacting on young people's mental and emotional health. These include:

Having a long-term physical illness: This is discussed in Chapter 6, where we focus on the vulnerabilities associated with chronic disease and illness, and other forms of physical, sensory and intellectual impairment.

Having a parent who has mental health problems, problems with alcohol or has been in trouble with the law: The stresses, difficulties and traumas of living with parents affected by these factors can be a major challenge to the mental and emotional health of a child or young person. Genetic influences can feature as a particular risk factor here, as a genetic propensity to develop some forms of mental illness, such as schizophrenia or depression, and addictive behaviours, such as alcoholism, can be inherited. Whether this propensity actually manifests itself in a young person can depend on their exposure to environmental stresses, however, including, unfortunately, exactly those that can arise in the chaotic environment created by this kind of situation. A pernicious vicious circle can develop leading to similar problems manifesting themselves in families across generations. Responses should involve interventions which address the needs of both the young person and the parent, and focus particularly on relieving the pressure of dealing with the situation from the young person. This is the kind of scenario where going into some form of care, either temporarily or permanently, may well be the best solution, although this is unlikely to happen without some form of crisis developing first. Options here would include local authority care (either provided directly or by a contracted organization) or foster care. A multi-agency approach involving Social Services, Health and Education will be needed, and an assessment of the young person by Child Adolescent Mental Health Services (CAMHs) should be a priority.

Experiencing the death of someone close to them: Bereavement is a natural part of the life cycle, and it is traumatic whenever it occurs. For it to occur in childhood or adolescence can add layers of complexity to the bereavement process, however, depending on the nature and circumstances of the death. The death of grandparents is perhaps the bereavement experience most to be expected. But just because it is 'expected' shouldn't diminish its possible impact, especially if the relationship was with a grandparent who played a major role in bringing the young person up as an infant and/or young child – not an uncommon scenario in the UK, where grandparents often provide childcare support to working parents. The death of a parent, sibling or close friend is also likely to have a major traumatic impact. The needs of the young person in this situation will centre on sensitive support to help them make sense of what has happened, and to grieve in a way that allows them to express and work through their emotions to a point where they can integrate the experience into their wider life narrative, allowing them to overcome possible feelings of guilt or injustice. This support may come from within the family network, but for adolescents, whose centre of gravity is naturally shifting away from the family, there may also be a need for support from outside – maybe from a trusted teacher, youth worker or group of friends. Identifying and accessing that source of support may well be the most crucial factor in helping a young person deal with bereavement.

Having parents who separate or divorce: With more than one in three marriages ending in divorce in the UK this has become an issue facing an increasing number of children and young people. Approximately 26 per cent of 10- to 19-year-olds now live in families with a lone parent. Not all of these are doing so because of divorce, of course, but a substantial proportion are. In 2011 it was estimated, for example, that nearly 38,000 of the 11- to 15-year-olds had parents who had divorced (Hagell et al., 2013). And that is likely to be an underestimate, as parents can also split up, of course, if they are cohabiting rather than legally married. As a risk factor the impact of parental divorce and separation is a complex one, and a great deal depends on the way the parents handle themselves and interact with each other in the process. Parental separation can actually be a good thing for young people's health and well-being if it brings to an end a period of conflict. And evidence also suggests that parents who are separating, or separated, will best address their children's psychological and emotional health needs if they actively help them to maintain their relationship with the other parent (Carr, 2004). Of course the circumstances leading to the split between parents may make this extremely difficult, but all the evidence suggests that parents who make the effort to put the emotional needs of their children first will see the best outcomes for them in the long term. Family therapy or mediation may be a potential option here, creating an independent space where the young person can have their perspective aired and responded to. A young person's needs in this situation may well be similar to those discussed above in relation to bereavement, and what was said there may also apply here – with the obvious difference that they may well need to maintain a relationship with the parent who is no longer around all the time, and may thus need ongoing and changing levels of support to do so.

Having been severely bullied or physically or sexually abused: Bullying and abuse – whether by a parent, other family member or from outside the family, up to and including organized crime – are serious threats to a young person's mental and emotional health and should be responded to as such. Young people themselves give bullying a high priority as an issue in their lives (ChildLine, 2008, cited in Roberts, 2012). Anxiety disorders, depression, post-traumatic stress disorder, self-harm and suicide and even the onset of schizophrenia, have all been linked to bullying and abuse (e.g. Roberts, O'Connor, Dunn and Golding 2004; Fisher, 2013; Moretti and Craig, 2013). A new dimension has been added in recent years with the advent of 'cyberbullying' via the internet and social networking sites, with an impact no less severe than that of face-to-face bullying. A recent survey by the anti-bullying charity 'Ditch the Label' (2013) found that seven out of ten young people – approximately 5.43 million – have experienced online bullying, with 23 per cent of those rating the abuse as extreme and occurring on a daily basis.

The most important intervention is to stop the bullying or abuse completely as quickly as possible and ensure that the young person is safe from further harm. Physical and/or sexual abuse is a child protection issue, and should be responded to immediately as such. This will involve removing the young person from the situation, and dealing with the perpetrators by sharing the appropriate information between service agencies – particularly Social Services and the Police – using formal multi-agency procedures (McCoglan, Campbell and Marshall, 2013). Beyond that, the young person's mental and emotional health needs will need to be properly assessed and monitored, with treatment and support provided as appropriate by specialist clinical services. The longer term care and support needs of an affected young person will also need to be addressed.

With bullying, the issues and responses may be more complex, but the same priority needs to be given to the young person's immediate safety and assessment of mental and emotional health needs. The nature and sources of the bullying need to be identified and responded to formally – by schools, for example – and it is important that the bully, and not the victim, is removed from the situation of contact. It is not unusual to find that the perpetrators of bullying are themselves victims of abuse or bullying, and that may well lead on to further levels of intervention. The young person affected by bullying needs to feel, however, that the people and institutional systems surrounding them are on *their* side, and committed to protecting them. The longer term mental and emotional health, well-being and safety of the affected young person will need to be addressed by ongoing collaboration between service agencies, professionals and the family.

Living in poverty or being homeless: This is of increasing importance in the current era of austerity. After a decade in which child poverty fell in the UK we have begun to see it rise again since 2010. Recent figures suggest that more than a fifth of 11- to 15-year-olds in the UK, some 22 per cent, live in families with the lowest incomes (Hagell et al., 2013). Poverty increases the likelihood of many of the other risk factors highlighted in this list, including abuse, parental mental illness and/or alcohol and substance abuse, and family breakdown. As such, the mental and emotional health issues faced by a young person will often be as discussed in relation to those factors.

Homelessness is one of the most extreme consequences of family breakdown, and the most extreme cause of poverty for a young person. Homelessness may itself be an outcome of trying to deal with mental and emotional health problems without proper support, or it may precipitate mental and emotional health problems. Whichever is the case, the main priority must be to get the young person off the streets and into a safe and supportive environment as soon as possible, and to assess and respond to the young person's mental and emotional health state.

Even where such extreme factors are not in play, poverty can have a corrosive effect on the mental and emotional well-being of young people. The rise of the consumer society in recent decades has helped to link young people's self-esteem and sense of identity to possessions – clothing and fashion, computer and smart phone technology, cars and motorbikes, for instance – that are the outward manifestations of wealth and status. This has been actively fuelled by a mass of corporate marketing aimed directly at young people, much of it designed precisely to provoke insecurities about their self-evaluation in comparison to others. This feeds into an innate human tendency to compare and judge ourselves in relation to other groups or individuals who we use as 'reference' points in, for example, appearance, wealth, possessions or sexual success – comparisons that can have a significant impact on self-esteem. It is important that young people use 'realistic' reference points for such comparisons, setting goals and standards consistent with their actual abilities and available resources (Carr, 2004). Consumer culture is largely built on promoting unrealistic comparisons, however, with advertising and marketing campaigns often setting up false and manipulated images for people to compare themselves against, particularly in terms of appearance. The anxiety and unhappiness provoked by this has been described by the psychotherapist Oliver James (2007) as 'affluenza' and part of the price we pay to live in consumer societies – more people who are miserable, self-absorbed and narcissistic. It has also been identified as one of the main causes of poor mental and emotional health in young people as they become increasingly obsessed by comparisons with others, particularly so-called celebrities.

Responding to this issue is highly problematic. For those working with and supporting young people, an overriding emphasis has to be placed on promoting their self-esteem and confidence in themselves, with reference to realistic and positive models for comparison. Many young people work out for themselves quite quickly how advertising and marketing embellishes and distorts reality, but many do not. And even those who do may still be left with a niggling feeling that they are somehow 'failing' if they are unable to acquire the latest smart phone or trainers. Some might argue that there is nothing wrong with this, and that it encourages aspiration and the motivation to study and work hard to attain 'success' and its trappings. Alternatively, it can be argued that it is both morally and psychologically corrupting to create a society full of what American poet and philosopher Gary Snyder has described as 'frustrated personalities' (Snyder, 1961). The authors here would argue that this is one of the big questions that those with power and influence in our society need to address, and it is an issue for health promotion at the national, political and institutional, as well as the personal, level, a point we will return to below.

Experiencing discrimination, perhaps because of their race, sexuality, disability or religion: The first thing to say about discrimination – that is, unfair, insulting or degrading treatment on the basis of race, religion, gender, sexuality or disability – is that it is illegal and can, and should, be reported to the authorities. That is easier said than done for some young people, however, particularly if their experience of the authorities is also one of discrimination. Young black men, for example, continue to experience discrimination from the police in some areas, being far more likely to be stopped and searched randomly (Dodd, 2013). And sometimes the authorities don't respond to protect the young person, even when hate crimes and harassment are reported. Quarmby (2011) has catalogued a disturbing litany of hate crimes against disabled people in the UK that the police and other authorities have often failed, or been very slow, to respond to appropriately – sometimes with fatal consequences.

There are strong parallels between issues of discrimination and those of bullying and abuse – and discrimination should be viewed as a form of both. Much of what was said about bullying and abuse applies here, therefore, and the priority is to focus on stopping it, protecting the young person from the discriminatory behaviour and removing them from harm's way. The point made about the young person feeling that the authorities and institutions are on *their* side is also relevant here. The impact on the affected young person's mental and emotional health will need to be assessed as a priority. Whatever this is, however, their capacity to survive, recover from and respond to experiences of discrimination will be greatly enhanced by sensitive and positive support from individuals and institutions.

Acting as a carer for a relative, particularly when it involves taking on adult responsibilities prematurely: Roles and responsibilities in families can sometimes be reversed, and many children and young people manage being a carer for one, and sometimes even both, parent(s) amazingly well. This should not blind us to the fact that some do not, however, and even those who do will need support to ensure their mental and emotional health is not compromised. The Young Minds Charity (2013) highlights the many difficulties and challenges faced by young carers, including managing the physical and psychological demands of caring whilst also trying to manage schoolwork and/or the transition to working adulthood. Opportunities to rest, relax, socialize and enjoy themselves – all important for young people's mental and emotional health and well-being – may be limited or absent altogether. They may also feel torn between feelings of resentment and anger about their situation and feelings of guilt about feeling such emotions.

Unsurprisingly, young people in this situation are at increased risk of developing mental and emotional health, and/or behavioural, problems. Support for young people in this situation has grown in recent years, with the establishment of 'Young Carers Groups' and youth counselling services in many areas. The critical factor is that someone, perhaps a teacher or neighbour, becomes aware of their situation and reports it to Social Services or, alternatively, the health team supporting the parent. Once again, assessment of the young person's mental and emotional health state is important, as is the involvement of a social worker to support the family.

Having long-standing educational difficulties: The term 'educational difficulties' covers a wide range of issues and risk factors, including most of those discussed above. Further risk factors can arise from having some form of neurologically rooted learning difficulty. The impact of more severe intellectual disabilities (learning difficulties) is discussed in Chapter 6.

So-called specific learning difficulties, such as dyslexia, dyscalculia or dyspraxia, may also be a risk factor, however. As the term suggests, these conditions tend to affect specific areas of cognitive performance rather than general intellectual functioning. The difficulties they give rise to may have a negative impact on the mental and emotional health of a young person, especially if they are either not detected and recognized, or the person is made to feel stupid, incompetent or inadequate by adults and peers around them (Selikowitz, 2004). The critical factors in response centre on identifying the problem and getting it properly assessed and 'officially' recognized, and then ensuring that targeted educational support follows. Assessment is usually carried out by an educational psychologist, and can be requested through the young person's school or paid for privately. The mental and emotional impact on the young person should also be assessed, and counselling support and/or advice given to help them understand the nature of the problem they are experiencing, and particularly that it is not their fault that they find certain areas of performance difficult. Educational support should also separate the particular area of difficulty the young person experiences – learning to read, write, understand maths or perform physical tasks – from other aspects of their learning. For example, their understanding of and enjoyment of subjects like history, geography or science, should be supported by scribes, 'speaking' computer programmes or apps, and alternative teaching methods and media, so that they are able to succeed educationally despite their specific difficulty. Accessing this kind of support often requires persistence and sheer 'bloody-mindedness' by a parent or advocate. As the authors know from personal experience, however, it should nonetheless be pursued, along with the determination to not take no for an answer!

Acute mental health problems

Emotional and mental health problems may lead into, or be an indication of, an acute mental health disorder such as schizophrenia, bipolar disorder, personality disorder or depression. Bailey and Shooter (2010) identify a number of acute mental health problems that need to be responded to as a matter of urgency, including:

- Depression in its various forms – bipolar, clinical, bereavement related, etc.

- Anxiety disorders – obsessive compulsive disorder (OCD), panic attacks, social phobias, etc.

- Post-traumatic stress disorder (PTSD)

- Eating disorders – anorexia nervosa and bulimia nervosa

- Self-harm

- Psychoses – schizophrenia

It is estimated that around half of all serious psychiatric disorders begin to manifest by age 14, and three quarters by age 24 (Hagell et al., 2013). It is critical that the condition is identified early and responded to appropriately by mental health services, although it is frequently other professionals and adults, particularly teachers and parents, who are likely to spot problems first. These will often manifest themselves in problematic or unusual behaviours at school or home. This highlights the need for teachers, youth workers and others to be aware of possible signs and symptoms, and to know who to share information with, particularly if the capacity of the young person's family to initiate this is limited or not possible.

The initial point of formal service contact and support will often be the young person's GP, school nurse or social worker. Onward referral to Child and Adolescent Mental Health services (CAMHs) is essential however. CAMHs departments are designed to provide dedicated mental health service coverage for children and young people, and were developed in recognition of the fact that, historically, provision for young people had often been patchy and of varying quality. The development of CAMHs ensured, for example, that mental health services addressed issues of accessibility and the appropriateness of settings – an issue highlighted by Vostanis (2007) as a critical factor in encouraging young people to access and maintain contact with services and treatments. As Vostanis points out, young people were often channelled into adult services and facilities that many found frightening, dangerous and stigmatizing. Unsurprisingly, this could lead to problems with subsequent attendance and treatment compliance, which in turn led some young people who desperately needed support and treatment to disengage from services altogether.

Acute mental health problems can be caused or precipitated by one or more of the risk factors listed above. PTSD, for example, an extreme form of anxiety disorder, can be caused by the traumatic experience of sexual or physical abuse or bullying. Such experiences are also known to be highly likely to cause or exacerbate severe depression and anxiety disorders such as OCD.

An association is also suspected between the onset of psychosis in some adolescents and some forms of substance use. There is a particular controversy surrounding the relationship between cannabis use and the onset of psychotic illness. The evidence is currently inconclusive as to whether this is a universal risk of cannabis use during the sensitive brain development phase of adolescence (particularly with high strength forms of cannabis such as 'skunk'), or whether cannabis use may act as a precipitator in some young people who are already at higher risk of developing psychosis due to underlying genetic factors. Some other psychoactive substances, including LSD and alcohol, have also been shown to precipitate psychotic illness in some people, with onset often occurring in late adolescence or early adulthood (Pycroft, 2010). The relationship between substance use and young people's health is discussed more fully in Chapter 9.

Treatments provided for acute mental illness need to be those recommended by the most reliable evidence-based practice, based on expert professional diagnosis by a clinical psychiatrist. Bailey and Shooter (2009) provide a valuable, plain language summary of the main treatments, including:

- **Talking therapies** – such as Cognitive Behaviour Therapy (CBT) – recommended to treat depression, anxiety disorders, social phobias and OCD;

- **Medications** – particularly anti-psychotics, anti-depressants and mood stabilizers, the use of which needs to be very carefully managed and monitored;

- **Complementary therapies** – such as omega3 fish oils and St John's Wort – which also need to be carefully managed and monitored.

To reiterate, acute mental health problems *must* be responded to by specialist mental health services and professionals, and an early referral to CAMHs is essential.

A wider response to the mental and emotional health needs of young people

It is important to recognize that a young person who experiences mental and emotional turmoil as a result of dealing with one or a mix of the risk factors discussed above is actually responding normally – not abnormally. Carr (2004) points out that depression, anxiety and anger are all important human emotions which have evolved to help us, paradoxically perhaps, to become happier and learn how to manage difficult situations and problems. Depression, for instance, teaches us to avoid or cope with distress, whilst anxiety teaches us to control or cope with fear, and anger teaches us to control our reactions to threats. All can become debilitating, however, when they take over our lives and rule our behaviour; and an inability to manage them can become a major obstacle to health, happiness and well-being.

Young people are, it seems, naturally disposed to be happy and optimistic. Hagell et al. (2013), reviewing recent research, highlight that four out of five young people report high life satisfaction, and the 16–19 age group is the most optimistic of all when questioned about prospects for the coming year. We also know that the capacity of a young person to recover from, or learn to manage, the problems they face very much depends on their level of resilience; a mixture, as we saw earlier, of their own internal resources (genetic factors and aspects of physical health, for instance) and protective factors related to the presence of external sources of support.

Coleman (2005) summarizes a range of research that emphasizes the importance of the presence of at least one supportive adult in helping a young person through a difficult time or experience. This emphasizes the point that resilience should be viewed not as a quality of 'strong' individuals – thereby implying that those who do not show high levels of resilience are weak – but as a *propensity* that can be nurtured in all young people with support. Expecting young people to deal with major life problems and traumas without access to such support is equivalent to adding the burden of taking on an 'adult level of responsibility' – itself a recognized risk factor – on top of whatever other problems and issues they may be facing. Ultimately, it should be seen as a form of neglect, by social institutions, communities and governments, every bit as much as by individual adults.

Vostanis (2007) makes the critical point that responding to the mental health needs of young people should be the responsibility of the whole community, with health services working collaboratively with families and schools in particular. He also echoes the point made elsewhere, that a proactive and preventative approach to promoting mental health in young people is far more cost effective, as well as morally sound, than waiting for problems to become acute and then mopping up the damage with expensive treatments or penal responses in years to come. Given the increasing problems with mental and emotional health and well-being faced by young people in the UK the main task facing concerned adults at all levels must be to increase their sensitivity and competence in responding to the psychological needs of young people. We would like to conclude this chapter, therefore, by emphasizing the need to focus on the wider social and cultural dimensions relating to young people's mental and emotional health and well-being.

Social and cultural factors

Writers and researchers, such as James (2007), Gerhardt (2010), Wilkinson and Pickett (2010), Dorling (2011) and Roberts (2012), have looked at, and sometimes compared, different social and cultural contexts and discussed the implications for the mental and emotional health of children, young people and indeed whole populations. A common theme that arises from the work of these authors is the clear relationship between declining mental and emotional health and the rise of selfish individualism and inequality that is a feature of modern capitalist societies like the UK.

In a similar vein, a series of recent reports, some of them government sponsored and commissioned, highlight the impact on the psychosocial health and well-being of children and young people of screen-based technologies and the internet (Byron, 2008); the sexualization of children and young people (Papadopoulos, 2011); the commercialization of childhood (Bailey, 2010); and the impact of inequality and materialism on children and young people's well-being (Nairn, 2011). The findings of these reports are discussed in more detail in other chapters, but they can perhaps be regarded also as discussions of particular symptoms of the more general malady identified by the authors above. And there are many echoes here too of the arguments in Chapter 4, made by Louv (2005), Palmer (2006) and Greenfield (2009).

Although the literature cited can be seen to represent widespread consensus regarding the problem, no such consensus seems to exist at the present time as to the solution. Debates continue about whether this lies with the voluntary, self-regulation of industries and corporations involved in areas such as fashion, computer gaming, alcohol advertising and internet and social media providers; or with parents who need to be much more aware and strict in their control of their children and teenagers; or governments, as the representatives and guardians of the health and well-being of their populations. We would argue, however, that the evidence as it stands, set out most fully by Wilkinson and Pickett (2010) in their comprehensive review of a wide range of indicators across the world's most affluent societies, strongly suggests that governments need to take the lead role – particularly in regulating the commercially driven agendas of large, hugely wealthy and politically influential corporations and marketing companies. The commercial imperatives of these organizations mean that they are highly unlikely to act voluntarily in ways which they would see as reducing their competitive edge. And the US child psychologist Susan Linn (2004) pointed out a decade ago that overworked and overstressed parents are unable to match the massive resources and relentless marketing machines of giant corporations.

The political consensus of 'deregulation' and unfettered commercialism that has dominated Western societies in recent decades is actually, all the evidence cited above indicates, what lies at the back of all of the critical social and cultural changes that are currently undermining the health and well-being of young people. We believe that a new evidence-based political consensus needs to be developed that challenges those mantras and places the highest value on the health and well-being of children and young people instead. The mental and emotional health of young people cannot be addressed by clinical and medical response systems alone, and, in many ways, to do so is to choose the most inefficient, least cost-effective and most morally questionable way of responding to their mental and emotional health needs. We will return to this argument in Chapter 10, but increasingly it is becoming clear that change at the political level is what is ultimately needed to address this issue.

Suggested Further Reading

Bailey, S. and Shooter, M. (2009) *The Young Mind: An Essential Guide to Mental Health for Young Adults, Parents and Teachers.* London: Royal College of Psychiatrists.
Bainbridge, D. (2009) *Teenagers: A Natural History.* London: Portobello Books.
Hagell, A. (2012) *Changing Adolescence: Social Trends and Mental Health.* Bristol: Policy Press.
Vostanis, P. (2007) Mental health and mental disorders. In J. Coleman and A. Hagell (eds), *Adolescence, Risk and Resilience: Against the Odds.* Chichester: John Wiley & Sons., pp. 89–106.
Weare, K. (2005) Taking a positive, holistic, approach to the mental and emotional health and well-being of children and young people. In C. Newnes and N. Radcliffe (eds) *Making and Breaking Children's Lives.* Ross-on-Wye: PCCS Books, pp. 115–122.

6

DISABILITY AND HEALTH IN YOUNG PEOPLE

In this chapter we will focus on some groups of young people who are more vulnerable to health problems than most. Newman (2004) defines vulnerability as, '… a feature that renders a person more susceptible to a threat' (p. 3). The groups of young people we will consider here can all be described as having such a feature, although we will argue that, often, it is not the 'feature' itself but the response of wider society to that feature that constitutes the main threat to their health and well-being. The groups we will focus on are those usually considered under the broad category of 'disability', including:

- **Learning difficulties (Intellectual impairment)** – that is, young people with impairments affecting global, rather than specific, aspects of intellectual functioning; also referred to under the terms 'learning disability' in UK policy, or 'intellectual disability' by the World Health Organization (the term 'impairment' is preferred here for reasons explained below). There are estimated to be some 286,000 children and young people (0–17) with learning difficulties in the UK, with around 200,000 having recognized special educational needs. Around four out of five are classified as having 'moderate' learning difficulties, and one in ten as having 'profound' learning difficulties. Moderate and severe learning difficulties have been identified as more common in some communities, including the traveller community, whilst profound multiple learning difficulties are more common in the Pakistani and Bangladeshi communities (Grant et al., 2010). Young people with acquired brain injury due to trauma or disease which occurs within the developmental period may also fall into this category.

- **Neuro-developmental disability** – is a term used sometimes as a broad 'catch-all' classification covering a wide range of the different groups (e.g. Blackburn, Read and Spencer, 2012). We use the term here in a more focused way, however, to refer to young people who have neurological conditions which mainly affect social functioning, communication and sometimes, but not always, wider intellectual functioning. These conditions include so-called high-functioning autistic spectrum conditions (ASC), attention deficit conditions, usually described as Attention Deficit Disorder (ADD), sometimes with hyperactivity (ADHD), and Tourette's syndrome. A significant rise in incidence has been noted in recent decades in all of these conditions, and they now constitute the largest group of disabled children and young people, with a total estimated prevalence for all conditions estimated at between 3 and 4 per cent of the population in the UK. The most commonly diagnosed condition, ADHD, is estimated to affect up to 2 per cent of children and young people, whilst around 1 per cent are affected by ASC (Blackburn, Read and Spencer, 2012). The prevalence of Tourette's syndrome is more difficult to specify, as the characteristics are often masked by its frequent co-occurrence with ASC and ADHD. The NHS Choices website (2014) suggests, however, that it may affect up to 1 in 100 children and young people.

Some commentators argue that the increase in prevalence is down to an increased tendency in the UK and elsewhere to pathologize behavioural problems that are actually rooted in overly regimented educational systems, the decline of 'natural play' in childhood and the rise of screen- and computer-based entertainments (e.g. Newnes and Radcliffe, 2005). This controversy will be discussed further below. It is widely agreed, however, that these conditions are often associated with emotional, behavioural and mental health problems. Young people with ASC, for example, are at higher risk of developing anxiety disorders, obsessive compulsive disorder (OCD) and depressive illness as they struggle to fit into social and educational environments which often fail to cater for their difference in learning and communication style or pace (Attwood, 2008).

- **Sensory disability** – that is, young people with visual and/or auditory impairments, occurring sometimes from birth, due, for example, to perinatal brain damage, abnormal development of the optic nerve or retina, or sometimes 'acquired' as a result of disease or trauma. There are estimated to be around 25,000 blind or partially sighted children in the UK – 2 in every 1000 – about half of whom also have a co-occurring physical or intellectual impairment. Young people with learning difficulties, for example, are ten times more likely to have a visual impairment than the general population (actionforblindpeople.org.uk, 2014). Also, there are around 45,000 hearing impaired children in the UK, most of whom are deaf from birth as a result of abnormal neurological or auditory nerve development (actionforhearingloss.org.uk, 2014).

- **Physical disability** – by which we mean young people with impairments affecting movement or functioning of the limbs and/or skeleton and muscle tone or strength, including both 'acquired' impairments (caused by accident or disease), or arising from congenital factors during development. It is surprisingly difficult to find separate statistics for young people with physical impairments. Most available statistics conflate physical and sensory impairments, for example, and some include it within even broader categories. One of the commonest conditions causing impairments of mobility, however, is Cerebral Palsy (CP), which is actually a range of conditions affecting about 1 in every 400 children (SCOPE Website, 2014). The impact of CP is highly variable, however, and can include a range of learning difficulties and sensory impairment as well. So, once again, the numbers get 'mixed-up' with those for other conditions.

- **Long-term, or 'chronic' health conditions** – by which we mean young people affected by conditions which cause long-term, sometimes life-long, and sometimes life-limiting, health problems – such as Type 1, or insulin-dependent, Diabetes, Asthma or Cystic Fybrosis. A term sometimes used to refer to young people affected by the need for long-term, sometimes intensive, medical and healthcare support to help them manage their lives is 'complex health needs'. This covers a vast range of conditions which can sometimes, but by no means always, co-occur with learning difficulties, neuro-developmental conditions and other physical or sensory impairments. The range of conditions which might fall under this category, and the potential mix with other categories, make identifying overall numbers even more difficult. For clinical and service provision purposes, therefore, most are considered as discrete groups.

Accurately identifying how many young people are affected by all of the conditions outlined above is not easy. A good deal depends on whether milder forms of impairment, such as mild hearing loss, are included (Mooney, Owen and Statham, 2008). The reason the data is being collected, and who is collecting it, will also have an impact. Those collecting data for epidemiological, educational or clinical purposes, for instance, may well arrive at different figures than those collecting data to assess eligibility to access services and benefits. We are currently seeing a significant and highly controversial shifting of the criteria for eligibility for accessing services and benefits for disabled people by both local and national government as part of the so-called austerity agenda. Blackburn, Read and Spencer (2012) give an overall figure of 0.8 million children and young people classified as disabled in the UK, around 6 per cent of all people under 18, but also argue that there is a need for more robust data, 'on the numbers, characteristics and circumstances' of disabled young people to inform service commissioners and policy makers (Davies 2012, Chapter 9, p. 11).

Causes and range of conditions

There are a huge range and diversity of causes of the impairments and conditions identified above. These include:

- *Biological (genetic/disease/developmental) causes* – recent surveys identify somewhere in the region of 7000 known genetically related conditions which may cause impairments or chronic illness (CAF Directory, 2013). And although infectious disease is no longer as prevalent as in previous historical eras, it is still a causative factor of some long-term conditions – brain damage caused by childhood meningitis, for instance. The negative effects of parental behaviours, although arguably 'social' rather than 'biological' in nature, can also be included here as they can have important impacts on foetal development. The impact of smoking, alcohol and/or substance abuse during pregnancy are all risk factors for premature birth, low birth weight or direct damage to the developing brain and central nervous system – as in foetal alcohol syndrome, for instance (Blackburn, Read and Spencer, 2012).

- *Accidents* – road traffic accidents are a significant cause of serious injury, including physical and/or brain damage, in the UK – particularly for young men (Dorling, 2011). Adolescence is a life stage associated with risky experimentation and, sometimes, miscalculation of risk. Other 'accidental' causative factors include poisoning (due mainly to alcohol or substance misuse), and spinal injury and/or near-drowning due to the miscalculation of risks whilst swimming or diving.

- *Head injuries and brain damage* – this can obviously be related to accidents, but may also occur as a result of physical abuse and violence, war and conflict, and some diseases, such as meningitis; or the various forms of epilepsy, often related to other causes and conditions – young people with ASC, for example, are up to five times more likely to develop epilepsy (Frith, 2008). And although the UK has not suffered the direct effect of being attacked for over 60 years (apart from thankfully rare terrorist attacks) our involvement in a number of conflicts in countries like Iraq and Afghanistan has led to a steady stream of war injured and traumatized young men and women attempting to return to normal life. Injury related to street violence, often related to excessive alcohol consumption, or gang-related violence is also a cause of various kinds of impairment – although there is some evidence that this type of violence has declined in recent years in the UK and across western Europe as a whole (Stengard and Appelqvist-Schmidlechner, 2010).

- *The effects of social deprivation and poverty* – poor diet, inadequate housing, unsafe and polluted environments, maternal smoking, alcohol and/or substance use during pregnancy, long-term unemployment and a lack of, or chaotic, family support are all implicated in poor physical and mental health outcomes for young people. And all of the factors highlighted in the sections above, from infectious disease to accidents and violence, are more likely to impact on young people from poorer communities. Poverty itself can be identified as *the* single most important cause of child and adolescent disability and poor health in the UK (Blackburn, Read and Spencer, 2012; Dorling, 2011; Roberts, 2012).

Conceptualizing and defining impairment and disability

In categorizing the various kinds of impairment that may affect young people it is easy to assume that our understanding of what disability is, and how we should respond to it, is not especially controversial. For much of the twentieth century the idea that disability in its various forms was a purely biomedical phenomenon, equivalent in most respects to disease and thus in need of similar programmes of eradication and treatment, went unquestioned; and to some extent this 'medical model' proved highly effective. Twentieth-century vaccination programmes very successfully eradicated or reduced the incidence of conditions such as Polio and Rubella, contracted during pregnancy, across the developed world – and attempts continue to extend that success across the developing world (Wolfe, 2011).

There are, however, a great many more forms of disability where the dominant role of the medical model has been questioned. The main challenge has come from politically active disabled people and their allies – the disability movement – who have developed the so-called social model of disability. The central tenet of the social model is the idea that the problems, or 'barriers', that disabled people face are more often due to living in a 'disabling society' – a society that largely fails to account for the needs of people with physical, sensory or intellectual impairments – than the actual impairments themselves. 'Disability' is redefined from this perspective as a category of social oppression, in a similar way to that associated with the categories of gender, race and sexual orientation (Oliver, 1996).

Although controversy remains as to the extent to which the social model has actually influenced policy and practice towards disabled people in the UK (e.g. Oliver and Barnes, 2012), Blackburn et al. (2012) point out that there has been a significant change in the way that disability has been conceptualized and responded to in recent decades. They argue that it is now widely accepted that attempts to improve the situation of disabled young people and their families must address the dynamic interrelationship between the young person's individual condition, and the physical, psychosocial and political/economic environment in which they live. In practice, this requires a threefold approach to responding to the needs of disabled young people.

First, it is important to recognize the **'impact of the impairment'** that the individual young person is experiencing. Supporting that young person will require that human service workers, be they medical, health, education, youth work and so on, have an awareness of the health-related characteristics of particular conditions, such as Downs' syndrome or ASC (both discussed as examples below), *and* a focus on how that condition impacts on the individual they are supporting. This may well include access to, and use of, medical and healthcare support, and it is important to grasp that an approach based on a social model of disability does not deny the importance of medical support and input – only that this should be appropriate and proportionate, rather than the totality of the response.

Second – and the main innovation that derives from the social model of disability – we also need to assess, identify and challenge the **'disabling barriers'** facing the young people we support. This brings ethical, legal, political and economic dimensions to the fore in the way that support is organized and delivered. It also requires critical examination of professional practice and support systems, and of the sociocultural and physical environments which disabled young people have to negotiate. This is by no means a secondary aspect in supporting young disabled people. As we shall explore further below, the disabling barriers – or disabilism – that many young disabled people confront can have a more serious impact on their lives than the impairment itself. As Goodley (2013) puts it; 'The psychological and emotional experience of disabilism is one subjected to everyday, mundane and relentless examples of cultural and relational violence' (p. 67).

Finally, support for disabled young people should be **'person-centred'** – that is, focused to as great an extent as possible on the individual needs, wishes and choices of the disabled young person themselves. Each young person affected by one, or a mix, of the conditions identified above will have an individual version and experience of that condition. In recent years we have seen a trend towards 'personalization' of care and support, including the individualization of budgets and self-directed support. This kind of model of service provision has been campaigned for by previous generations of disabled people, and has been pioneered in other parts of the world – particularly Scandinavia and North America. Some controversy surrounds the actual implementation and practice of these approaches, however, and there is a strong suspicion that cost-cutting agendas are an important undercurrent in the way this policy has been implemented by recent UK governments. Issues remain about the actual amounts of money available; restrictions on what it can be used for – and thus who is actually in control; unequal access to direct payments for certain groups such as people with learning difficulties, for instance; and the additional workload burden for individuals and families of managing budgets – effectively becoming an employer and manager of their own care and support packages. Nonetheless, the move towards more individualized and personalized models of care and support is generally seen as a positive move – and person-centredness is an important ethos for all those working with disabled young people (Franklin, 2013).

The threefold approach in practice

Having set out the threefold approach, we will now go on to explore what it may look like in practice, illustrating our discussion with some examples. The vast range of impairments that may affect young people makes it is impossible here to address all types, versions and permutations, so this will inevitably be a very generalized discussion, and we will stick to the general categories used above.

Intellectual impairment

The impact of intellectual impairment varies hugely across conditions and between individuals affected by the same condition. The main shared characteristic, however, is an impairment of learning and processing of information relating, for example, to the management of time, literacy, numeracy, self-organization, and the social and cultural appropriateness of various behaviours. This should not be taken to mean that an affected person is not able to learn and develop new knowledge and competencies – an attitude that constitutes a major disabling barrier – but that the extent to which they can do so lies outside the range considered normative for an individual to achieve social and economic autonomy, or manage independently, within mainstream work or educational environments.

The line defining 'normal' from 'abnormal' levels of functioning is, of course, all important here, and the issue of the classification of who does and who does not fall within the range defined as 'normal' makes this an area where we confront another significant disabling barrier – that classification systems of all forms of impairment in our society are used not just as biomedical and/or clinical descriptions to aid diagnosis, but also as criteria for deciding who can, and who cannot, access financial, educational and social support. Access to such support is vital to the health and well-being of young people with learning difficulties. Learning to lead a healthy lifestyle requires knowledge, social, cultural and economic opportunities, as well as access to quality relationships and environments. Denial of these opportunities is a serious disabling barrier and a failure of political will – not an inevitable outcome of having an intellectual impairment.

To illustrate the importance of assessing the impact of impairment on an individual, let us look at the example of Downs' syndrome:

Example 1: Downs' syndrome

Downs' syndrome is a genetic condition, most frequently, but not exclusively, caused by a chromosomal anomaly referred to by geneticists as 'trisomy 21', where an extra chromosome is translocated to the 21st pair of chromosomes. It is associated with variable degrees of intellectual impairment causing learning difficulties, ranging from moderate to severe. It is also frequently associated with a number of physiological characteristics which can compromise health and well-being, including:

- Cardiovascular abnormalities – which can be severe, and even life threatening

- Respiratory problems – associated with characteristically narrow respiratory openings and canals, such as the Eustachian tubes that connect the ear and mouth

- Musculatory and skeletal problems – particularly low muscle tone and spinal column weaknesses, especially around the join with the base of the skull

- Neurological problems – including early onset Alzheimer's disease in middle to late adulthood

- Endocrinological problems – such as thyroid problems.

An awareness of these characteristics and physiological factors means that we can proactively recognize and respond to potential risk factors to the physiological and psychological health and well-being of young people with Downs' syndrome. For example, given the possibility of cardiovascular, skeletal and respiratory problems, health education and support around maintaining a healthy diet and weight has particular importance in establishing good physiological health now and in later life. Regular monitoring and assessment of aspects of physiological health – such as annual assessment of thyroid functioning – is also important, as abnormal thyroid functioning can have serious implications for both weight gain and intellectual functioning.

Historically, 'care' systems for people with Downs' syndrome, and indeed people with learning difficulties generally, have not addressed these factors to the extent they should, often leading to preventable chronic ill health and early death. The promotion of good physical health, therefore, is very significant in promoting an optimum quality of life for young people with Downs' syndrome – and all young people with learning difficulties. Good physiological health also helps establish and maintain good psychological and emotional health and well-being, and helps to promote positive self-image and self-esteem.

Physical impairment

The impact of physical impairment will obviously depend on which aspects of physical functioning are affected. The most common functions affected are likely, however, to be related to mobility, which is often actually a problem of accessibility, and thus a disabling barrier related to environmental design factors, rather than an impact of impairment. Oliver (1993) has pointed out that the inability to walk is not necessarily a 'health' impact in itself, and can relatively easily be addressed using the increasingly sophisticated electric wheelchair and/ or prosthetic limb technology now available; and by focusing on redesigning buildings and the wider built environment to make them accessible.

However, it should also be remembered that the opportunity to work on and develop physical fitness can be important for young people with physical impairments. Achieving and maintaining optimum muscle tone and bone density may well be an issue that can help to optimize quality of life, and have beneficial psychological impacts on self-esteem. One of the positive legacies of the 2012 Paralympics in London was to illustrate that the capacity to develop high levels of physical fitness, skill and ability is by no means limited to the so-called able-bodied – although one could ask why the Paralympics has to exist as a separate event, and could not be included as part of a mainstream Olympics, which would then more accurately reflect the full range of human diversity?

The aspiration to attain highly athletic levels of physical fitness is not universal however, and there are many other reasons to promote optimum physical health for young people with physical impairments. A physically sedentary lifestyle can increase the risk of a variety of weight, dietary and digestive problems, all of which can lead to avoidable health problems in later life, including heightened risks of heart disease, bowel cancer and type 2 diabetes.

Example 2: Cerebral Palsy

In conditions like Cerebral Palsy (CP), where physical mobility may be restricted, and which may also affect a young person's capacity to maintain an upright posture, there are heightened risks of respiratory, digestive and skeletal problems, which can all lead to potentially serious health problems – such as an increased risk of developing pneumonia from a respiratory infection. Such problems may also cause extreme discomfort and chronic pain. Attention to accessing, maintaining and updating the best quality posture-supporting equipment, and issues of managing hygiene and continence, will therefore need to be addressed as priorities. Sensitive management of such issues is vital in promoting psychological and emotional, as well as physiological, health and well-being. The development of a positive self-image and high self-esteem are strongly linked to a sense of physical well-being, comfort and dignity – something acutely felt in adolescence. A key factor in ensuring success will be to build support systems around the active participation, and ideally control, of the young person themselves, to whatever extent they are able to manage. This will include, for example, choice and control over who, when, where and how support is delivered (Franklin, 2013) – a point that can be generalized to all of the categories of young people discussed here.

Sensory impairment

Health issues relating to sensory impairment will focus on maintaining safety, promoting communication and accessing support for opportunities to develop mobility, physical and psychological health and well-being. The capacity to travel safely around cities, communities and important buildings, such as schools, colleges, universities, workplaces and leisure facilities, is particularly important for young people with visual impairments. Much of the answer to this lies in designing and planning adjustments to the environment – such as lowered and textured pavements, 'talking' lifts and automatic doors. Features like this have been incorporated into some aspects of the environment for many years – 'Pelican Crossings', for example. Making environmental adjustments more generally available across social, cultural and institutional environments has involved a concerted political struggle, however, to persuade or legally enforce environmental planners, architects, corporate leaders, public service managers and politicians, at local, national and international levels, to recognize that not addressing this amounts to the construction of significant disabling barriers to people who have sensory and other forms of physical impairment.

Communication issues are also of huge importance for young people with sensory impairments. The key issue is to ensure that provision is made for young people with visual and hearing impairments to access the same level of social, educational and work opportunities open to all other young people. A failure to address the provision of braille, signing, audio/visual and personal assistant support, as appropriate, amounts to the serious disablement of young people with sensory impairments that is purely social in nature, and nothing to do with the impairment itself. And, as with all of the conditions referred to here, service provision and support should be seen as an economic, as well as a social, investment that will actually reduce costs over the longer term as those young people are supported to become empowered, autonomous and productive, rather than passively dependent.

Neuro-developmental conditions

As noted above, we appear to be witnessing significant increases in the incidence of conditions such as ASC, ADHD and Tourette's syndrome in the UK.

There has been much debate, much of it rather panic stricken and sensationalist in nature, as to what is happening and why. The main factor is undoubtedly an increased and more widespread knowledge and awareness of these conditions among parents, child care professionals and teachers. We are now far better at identifying young people with these conditions, whereas before they may have been missed completely or written off as merely being 'badly behaved' (King and Bearman, 2009). Silberman (2015) has described how the development and increasing sophistication of diagnostic tools, such as the Diagnostic and Statistical Manual (DSM) of the American Psychiatric Association, now in its 5th edition, has contributed to this; something deliberately campaigned for by pioneering researchers, particularly the late Lorna Wing, in order to ensure that more children and families could receive the diagnosis that would qualify them to access support and services. Other factors are at work too, however, including: changes in the psychosocial and cultural environment in which children and young people develop, including significant increases in computer games and screen-based entertainment; the decline of 'natural play' in natural environments; issues related to nutrition; and an increasingly regimented and competitive education system – all particularly implicated in the continuing rise of ADHD (e.g. Jackson, 2002; Timimi and Radcliffe, 2005).

- Genetic factors have also been identified in the inheritance of these conditions – although it is only as we have become more aware of these conditions in current cohorts of children that some parents have recognized them in themselves and their own family histories (Atwood, 2008).

- 'Over-diagnosis' – the flip side of an increased awareness and diagnosis is the tendency to 'pathologize' the behaviours of some children and young people who, it is argued, have learning styles not easily accommodated in the mainstream educational system (Silberman, 2015). There is continuing controversy, for example, about ADHD, with some researchers and commentators arguing that it is a condition largely 'invented' and promoted by psychiatry and the pharmaceutical industry. Certainly, the prescription of Ritalin as a response to behavioural problems has increased massively in the US in particular, and in the UK too (Brown, 2005).

The DSM (5) identifies sets of behavioural criteria for each condition. There is a considerable range of variation in the manifestation of characteristics in different individuals, however – so much so that it can be extremely hard to separate the different conditions out. Kutscher (2007) describes this as 'the syndrome mix' and argues that diagnosis is often based on the dominant characteristics as they manifest themselves in an individual, rather than a single 'classical' set of characteristics associated with one or other of the conditions. Thus a young person with traits associated with high-functioning autism will very probably also show traits associated with ADHD and/or Tourette's syndrome. If, however, it is 'autistic' characteristics that dominate, then the diagnosis of autism is the one that will be made. This is one of the reasons why a conclusive diagnosis can sometimes be hard to come by; and it also raises questions about the scientific validity of the diagnostic criteria being used. Despite these controversies, a diagnosis is nonetheless vital to, and welcomed by, many parents and affected young people themselves, as it is the main way in which important support and resources can be accessed.

Neuro-developmental conditions tend to manifest themselves in atypical behavioural and developmental patterns, or 'trajectories', in the young people they affect. Kutscher (2007) presents them as a group of conditions that have their basis in atypical development and functioning of the areas of the brain known as the frontal and pre-frontal cortex. These areas are strongly associated with 'executive functioning' – including self-organization and planning of behaviour, such as taking into account past experience, gauging possible consequences and outcomes, the ability to empathize with others and judge how others will perceive and respond to your behaviour. The main impact of these conditions, therefore, is often an impairment of social functioning, which tends to manifest itself as a more or less extreme form of social awkwardness, including:

- Difficulty in responding to and managing normal communication cues, such as appropriate levels of eye contact or appropriate spacing of conversational responses – taking longer to answer than normal, or 'butting in' with an abrupt change of subject, for example.

- Difficulty understanding the use of, or 'getting', humour, sarcasm or irony, all of which are significant resilience-related behaviours and ways of managing the day-to-day trials, tribulations and complexities of adolescent social life.

- Responding to others in an 'over-emotional' – particularly aggressive or anxious – way.

- Withdrawal from social contact into what are felt to be 'safe' environments, such as their bedroom; or repetitive routines and instantly gratifying and controllable activities, such as computer games.

Because other aspects of their intellectual functioning are often unaffected, the severity of the disabling impact of these social difficulties can be overlooked (Jackson, 2002). Young people affected by them are particularly vulnerable to social isolation, bullying and increased levels of social anxiety. This in turn places them at increased risk of developing mental and emotional health problems, including depression, anxiety disorders and Obsessive Compulsive Behaviours (Kutscher, 2007; Hendricx, 2010).

An added element of 'cultural risk' with neuro-developmental conditions is their physical invisibility and expression in primarily behavioural forms. In a culture dominated by an ideology of competitive individualism young people affected may be perceived effectively as weak, immature or even as lying in order to gain the benefits of a 'sick role' – namely opting out of the cultural obligation to work. This is another reason why a medical diagnosis, such as 'autism', may be welcomed by parents and affected individuals; so they can claim a legitimate disabled identity.

Example 3: Autistic Spectrum Condition (ASC)

The impact of ASC varies hugely, from profound levels of intellectual and communication impairment, to high, and sometimes exceptional, levels of intellectual functioning, although with difficulties in understanding and managing social situations and interactions. ASC is also associated with a number of mental health problems and issues. Young people with ASC are known, for example, to be at increased risk of developing depression, although the relationship is a complex one. The isolating nature of the impairment may play a part, but so too can the difficulties young people with ASC experience in coping with the complex social environment in which they find themselves, which can lead to heightened levels of stress and anxiety. This can become serious, developing into obsessive compulsive disorders (OCD), or social phobias, which can lead to further problems in managing school, college and other areas of life.

There is a strong interrelationship also between ASC and other neuro-developmental conditions, such as Tourette's syndrome. Young people with ASC frequently experience movement problems, either as part of their impairment or as a side effect of psychotropic medication – this can manifest itself sometimes as self-injurious behaviours (associated with Tourette's), and can also be associated with OCD (Kutscher, 2007). The promotion of relaxation techniques and the use and maintenance of 'safe' places and routines can all be used to help mitigate the effects of anxiety (Hendricx, 2010).

Autism has sometimes been confused in the past with schizophrenia, although co-occurrence is actually rare. Cases of both auditory and visual hallucination are known to occur, however. This is known as 'synaesthesia', a linking of the sensory areas of the brain that causes a stimulatory interreaction between the senses – 'hearing lights' and 'seeing noises', for example (Ramachandran, 2011). This may underlie some of the difficulties that young people with ASC have in managing certain loud and 'over-stimulating' environments and activities; and a stress response to sound, light, taste or other sensory stimuli – or even what looks like a fairly normal classroom environment – should lead to an investigation of this as a possibility. Synaesthesia should not always be regarded as a negative phenomenon, however. Ramachandran (2011) has shown it to be quite common among highly creative people, and some artists and musicians identify it as an important factor in their creativity (e.g. Hart, 1990).

Another remarkable feature present in some people with ASC is so-called savant abilities. This is where the person demonstrates an exceptional ability, or set of abilities, in isolated areas of functioning. Where this has artistic and commercial value it can be used to build a successful working life and career for the individual. An example of this in the UK is the artistic career of Stephen Wiltshire, whose capacity to draw detailed panoramas of buildings and cities has been used to help him become a highly successful commercial artist (Treffert, 2010).

Overall, efforts to sensitively engage young people with ASC in social and community life, education, leisure and work opportunities are very important, as is access to youth counselling and pastoral services (Hesmondhalgh and Breakey, 2001). And an important supportive approach that has been developed to help young people with high-functioning autism is 'signposting'. This is based on the idea that we need to understand how autism affects young people's thoughts, feelings and understanding of the world, so that we can respond to them as people who need answers to certain questions to feel safe and comfortable – these questions are:

- Where should I be?
- What do I have to do?
- When do I do it?
- How long will it last?
- Who do I do it with?

An important aim in working with young people with ASC is to negotiate, anticipate and answer these questions to help them make sense of what is happening and reduce any anxiety they may be feeling (Atwood, 2008).

A similar kind of approach can also be applied to young people more severely affected by autism, including those with associated severe, or even profound, learning difficulties. A number of specialized communication-based techniques and approaches, such as 'Intensive Interaction' (Hewett, Firth, Barber and Harrison, 2012) and the 'Sonrise' approach developed in the USA (Kaufman, 2014), have proved particularly valuable. These approaches emphasize teaching the value and rewards of communication and human relationships, often through play-based, interactive techniques. Although the scientific validity of the 'Sonrise' programme has been questioned, both approaches have a track record of reducing challenging and self-injurious behaviours, and improving the communication skills, confidence and quality of life of affected young people and their families.

Autistic spectrum conditions – an affirmative perspective

Some people with ASC who have higher levels of cognitive functioning have developed something of a different 'take' on their condition, seeing it as a positive identity, and even as a strength. They highlight, for example, the intense levels of concentration and focus that people with ASC can demonstrate – sometimes pathologized as 'obsessiveness' from a psychomedical perspective – but which can lead to the development of high levels of knowledge, skill and technical application in areas such as computer programming and information technology. An example is Temple Grandin, a professor of animal behaviour at the University of Colorado in the US, who has autism, and is a leading advocate for people with ASC. She has argued that autism has been a positive benefit to her in allowing her to understand the animal brain, and thus to design holding equipment which reduces stress and fear in farm animals in abattoirs and for veterinary procedures (Grandin and Panek, 2014).

'Aspies', as some people with high-functioning autism style themselves, have gone on to pioneer an affirmative view of themselves and those with other 'conditions' (including ADHD and Tourette's syndrome). They have sought to reconstruct a positive 'neurodiversity' approach to understanding and supporting people with ASC and other neuro-developmental conditions (e.g. Bloome, 1998; Hendrickx, 2010). They also challenge the negative and pathological view propagated by so-called neuro-typicals, and reflected in their dismay at the dropping of the Asperger's syndrome categorization in the DSM (5). It is likely that something of a battle will develop over this term that illustrates the contested nature of identity in this area.

Long-term and chronic health conditions

There are a huge variety of long-term and chronic conditions affecting the health and well-being of young people. A critical general principle for human service workers and professionals is to learn as much as they can about the condition affecting the young person they are supporting. Many of these conditions require regular, sometimes daily, and sometimes even continuous, monitoring and medical support in order to mitigate their impact. To illustrate this, we will look at the still relatively little known example of Cyclical Vomiting Syndrome (CVS).

Example 4: Cyclical Vomiting Syndrome (CVS)

CVS is a good example of one of the many lesser known genetically related conditions, where individuals are generally in good health, but can experience debilitating attacks and symptoms which are not always predictable in terms of onset and duration, although attacks can be linked to negative stress in some people. This can make this – and similar conditions – very difficult for a young person to manage and organize their life around.

CVS is a genetic condition whose actual causation is still not fully understood, but is thought to lie in a mutation of mitochondrial DNA. The main symptom of CVS is prolonged bouts of vomiting, accompanied by lethargy and persistent nausea. Vomiting can reach peaks of four to five times an hour and last for periods of hours, or even days, with an average duration of between 12 hours and 2 days. Onset of the condition is usually in middle childhood, and it can persist for years and possibly for life in some individuals. CVS is usually diagnosed after all other potential causes of nausea and vomiting have been eliminated, and, as yet, there is no specific test for diagnosis. The CVS Association website (2014) states that the condition appears to run in families, particularly where there is a family history of travel sickness and migraine, and refers to studies conducted in Australia and Scotland that suggest a prevalence of around 2 per cent in school age children.

Medical research is currently focused on trialling anti-emetic drugs as treatments, but no one drug has emerged, as yet, as a universal treatment. Treatment therefore focuses on caring and comforting support, helping the person to lie in a quiet, darkened and comfortable room, and maintaining fluid intake to avoid dehydration.

The psychological impact of managing a condition such as CVS also needs to be addressed, and we know from the examples of more common conditions, such as type 1 Diabetes, that affected young people benefit from counselling and pastoral support, and particularly support groups where they can meet and share knowledge and experiences with others who are also affected – and know they are not alone and that their experience is shared (e.g. Harris and Hall, 2014).

Perhaps the most significant requirement for a young person managing CVS – and this applies to many other conditions requiring ongoing medical and healthcare support – is that they have the time and space to manage symptoms, and receive treatments to mitigate their impact, without harming their educational and vocational development or employment chances. Whatever treatments may arise from medical research, young people with CVS will also need to have legally enforceable rights to ensure that they receive a guarantee of educational and vocational support to provide the same opportunities to achieve in education and employment as any other young person.

Some points of good practice

Some general principles of good practice for human service workers supporting disabled young people include:

- **Know your impairments** – find and make use of sources/resources that can help educate you, especially those written and created by young disabled people themselves and their families.

- **Regard the young person, and their parents and carers, as experts, partners and resources** – the affected young person is *the* most important resource you have in achieving a person-centred approach.

- **Educate yourself about the roles and identities of other professions and agencies who can help** – effective multi-agency and interprofessional working is essential in supporting young disabled people to access all the resources and support they need – cultivate good communication systems with all and create a 'collaborative culture' around them (Beresford and Trevillion, 1995).

- **Become an advocate for young disabled people** – argue and campaign for social, political and economic change. Work to break down disabling barriers, and become part of the 'culture of resistance' among disabled people and their allies, which we will explore further below.

Conclusion – understanding and confronting disabling barriers

Many of the problems that disabled young people face are related to the discriminatory, and sometimes directly oppressive, way that society responds to people with impairments – that is, 'disablism' – rather than the functional impairments they experience. Blackburn et al. (2012) highlight significant barriers to social participation compared with non-disabled young people. These include lack of money, poorly designed buildings, high streets, leisure, sport and workplaces, and transport systems which, despite the existence of anti-discriminatory legislation, are still often difficult to access. They can also include psychosocial barriers, including negative attitudes, stereotyping and discriminatory attitudes up to and including hate crime (Quarmby, 2011). Blackburn et al. (2012) also identify significant barriers to accessing services and support. In particular they highlight the frequent lack of coordination between agencies in many areas, and wide variations and inequalities in the provision of short-term breaks, direct payments and access to mental health and behavioural support.

In material terms, disabled young people are much more likely to be excluded from further and higher education, and from employment. It has been estimated that around 28 per cent of disabled children face significant barriers to accessing education, leisure and play. Poverty is an important factor, with household income for families with a disabled child some 13 per cent lower on average than families without a disabled child. Children and young people in socioeconomically disadvantaged households are twice as likely to develop a disability in later childhood. Disabled young people are also more likely to live in single parent families, and almost half of disabled children have parents who are themselves also disabled. Whilst there is no intrinsic reason why disabled young people cannot live fulfilling, healthy and happy lives, these disabling barriers mean that they are at greater risk of poor health, and also poor educational and employment outcomes (Blackburn et al., 2012).

Priestly (2013) argues that we need to take account of the life stage when examining disabling barriers. The adolescent life stage can be characterized as the transformation of identity from child to adult. In affluent, 'post-industrial' societies such as the UK, however, identity has become a much more fluid concept, mediated by more-or-less conscious consumer choices made within an open market place (Urry, 1990). A common experience of disabled young people, however, is exclusion from these so-called open markets and the choice-making options open to most young people. Significant parts of their identity are often constructed around them by a dominant 'medicalized' view of disability, associated with 'deeper' cultural images that associate disability with disease and deformity. Such images and 'identity markers' often run counter to those promoted and idealized in the market-dominated, consumerist social milieu in which most young people live. Youthful beauty, energy, mobility and agility are presented as desirable ideals and aspirations. This has troubling enough consequences for many able-bodied and able-minded young people. For many disabled young people it can amount to a near impenetrable wall of exclusion (Hughes, Russell and Paterson, 2005). Many young disabled people are acutely aware of these cultural processes of exclusion with important implications for their health and well-being, and their capacity for resilience (Morris, 2002). This has led to the emergence of what Brandon and Elliot (2008) have described as a 'culture of resistance' among disabled people, one manifestation of which is the affirmative model of disability.

The affirmative model of disability is particularly associated with the work of John Swain and Sally French (2008). They observe that, 'while tragedy [is] the dominant view of disability and impairment, the writings of disabled people [express] a far more varied and positive picture.' The affirmative model, they assert, '...is a way of thinking that directly challenges presumptions about the experiences, lifestyles and identities of people with impairments' (p. 65).

In an interview in the *New Scientist* magazine Professor Stephen Hawking, widely recognized as one of the world's leading scientists, and also affected by severe physical impairment due to the progression of a form of motor neurone disease, argues that his condition has been a blessing, allowing him to concentrate his energies on the intense intellectual activity that has made him one of the world's leading theoretical physicists (George, 2009). Although Professor Hawking has not himself, to our knowledge, formally advocated an affirmative model of disability, this quote could well be seen as an example of the affirmative model in action – the idea that the condition experienced by a disabled person is not seen as a tragedy or disaster, where they automatically assume a passive and dependent existence, living some kind of half-life that imitates, but can never capture, the fullness of normality. Instead, the condition is seen as allowing, or even liberating, the person to be more fully themselves – as a platform from which to make their own unique contribution to their own life, and to society as a whole. Other examples that could be cited are those of animal behaviour scientist Temple Grandin and commercial artist Stephen Wiltshire, both mentioned earlier in our discussion of ASC. And Brandon and Elliot (2008) cite a range of other less well known examples of artists, writers, musicians, theatre groups and other disabled activists all busy creating the 'culture of resistance'.

The focus on creating and celebrating a positive sense of identity for disabled people that is the hallmark of both the affirmative model of disability, and the neuro-diversity movement, is particularly relevant, we would argue, when looking at the situation of young disabled people. For previous generations of disabled people and their allies, the primary struggle was to reclaim access to mainstream society and its material benefits. That is a struggle that continues – and has intensified again recently as benefits and services for disabled people have been stripped away as part of the so-called austerity agenda. However, it is at the deeper level of cultural change that the struggle will ultimately be won, as young disabled people claim and celebrate their own identity, both individually and collectively – as have black people, gay people and other oppressed groups before them. And in doing so they will, ultimately, of course, enhance the quality of all our lives.

Suggested Further Reading

Armstrong, T. (2010) *The Power of Neurodiversity: Unleashing the Advantages of Your Differently Wired Brain*. Philadelphia: Da Capo Books.

Bailey, S. and Shooter, M. (2009) *The Young Mind: An Essential Guide to Mental Health for Young Adults, Parent and Teachers*. London: Royal College of Psychiatrists.

Blackburn, C., Read, J. and Spencer, N. (2012) Children with neurodevelopmental disabilities. In S. Davies, *Annual Report of the Chief Medical Officer 2012: Our Children Deserve Better*. London: HMSO.

Franklin, S. (2013) *Personalisation in Practice: Supporting Young People with Disabilities through the Transition to Adulthood*. London: Jessica Kingsley Publishers.

Hendrickx, S. (2010) *The Adolescent and Adult Neuro-diversity Handbook: Asperger Syndrome, ADHD, Dyslexia, Dyspraxia and Related Conditions*. London: Jessica Kingsley Publishers.

Jackson, L. (2002) *Freaks, Geeks and Asperger Syndrome: A User Guide to Adolescence*. London: Jessica Kingsley Publishers.

Oliver, M. and Barnes, C. (2012) *The New Politics of Disability*. Basingstoke: Palgrave Macmillan.

7
SEXUAL HEALTH AND YOUNG PEOPLE

In this chapter we will look at sexual health issues for young people and discuss some of the approaches and strategies used to address them. We will identify the key issues and explore what the evidence tells us about them. As a preliminary, however, we need to define some key terms and concepts to clarify what we mean when we talk about sexual well-being. The following definitions are taken from the World Health Organization Report of a Technical Consultation on Sexual Health 28–31 January 2002 (WHO, 2006).

- *Sex* – refers to the biological characteristics that define humans as female or male. While these sets of biological characteristics are not mutually exclusive – there are individuals who possess both – they tend to differentiate humans as males and females. The term 'sex' is also sometimes used to mean 'sexual activity', but for technical purposes in the context of sexuality and sexual health discussions, the above definition is preferred.

- *Sexuality* – is a central aspect of being human throughout life and encompasses sex, gender identities and roles, sexual orientation, eroticism, pleasure, intimacy and reproduction. Sexuality is experienced and expressed in thoughts, fantasies, desires, beliefs, attitudes, values, behaviours, practices, roles and relationships. While sexuality can include all of these dimensions, not all of them are always experienced or expressed. Sexuality is influenced by the interaction of biological, psychological, social, economic, political, cultural, ethical, legal, historical, religious and spiritual factors.

- *Sexual health* – is a state of physical, emotional, mental and social well-being in relation to sexuality; it is not merely the absence of disease, dysfunction or infirmity. Sexual health requires a positive and respectful approach to sexuality and sexual relationships, as well as the possibility of having pleasurable and safe sexual experiences, free of coercion, discrimination and violence. For sexual health to be attained and maintained, the sexual rights of all persons must be respected, protected and fulfilled.

- *Sexual rights* – embrace human rights that are already recognized in national laws, international human rights documents and other consensus statements.

They include the right of all persons, free of coercion, discrimination and violence, to:

- the highest attainable standard of sexual health, including access to sexual and reproductive health care services;
- seek, receive and impart information related to sexuality;
- sexuality education;
- respect for bodily integrity;
- choose their partner;
- decide to be sexually active or not;
- consensual sexual relations;
- consensual marriage;
- decide whether or not, and when, to have children;
- pursue a satisfying, safe and pleasurable sexual life.

In addition to the above, a very useful definition of sexual well-being for those working with young people is given on the Durex website:

> Sexual wellbeing is a balance of physical, emotional and sociological factors. It's about protecting and nurturing the sexual health of both you and your partner, getting the most from your sex life and feeling confident and happy about yourself. Sexual wellbeing is a fundamental part of human wellbeing and health.
>
> (www.durex.com)

Adults will speak to young people with ease about the benefits and pleasures of healthy eating, but are loath, it seems, to admit that the main reason many adults engage in sexual activity is to do with pleasure. And yet, as the 'Durex definition' illustrates, sexual well-being is arguably as important to human health and well-being as the nutritional quality of our food.

Sexuality and values

It is important also to remember how personal values can influence our approach and responses to the issues of young people's sexual health. In understanding how our own responses to the sexual health issues of young people have been shaped by our own upbringing, education, socialization and life experiences, we are better equipped to react in a measured and non-judgemental way when supporting young people.

From the moment we are born we experience the influence of families, friends, siblings, school, religion, television, music, media and the world around us. It is these experiences that help form our belief system, which may at first manifest itself as received wisdom, until we gradually learn the skills and self-awareness to adapt and develop our own beliefs. Ideally, the role of professionals working with young people – teachers, youth workers, health professionals or others – involves being able to give impartial, non-judgemental advice, information and guidance. To do that effectively involves being able to acknowledge and manage our own values and beliefs. Whilst we cannot, and should not be required to, deny our own belief systems, we should nonetheless be guided primarily by the needs of young people, rather than ourselves. It is not appropriate or helpful, for example, for professionals working with young people to present sexual health information that reflects their own cultural and/or religious beliefs if they run counter to the sexual rights as stated above. Practitioners must refrain from imposing their own belief systems, or personal views, when addressing sexual health issues with young people, and if they have difficulty in doing so, need to consider whether they are in the right role.

Healthy sexual development

To be sexually healthy requires, first, a positive approach to human sexuality, and an understanding of the complex mix of factors that shape human sexual behaviour. These factors may well determine whether a young person's expression of sexuality leads to sexual health and well-being, or places them more at risk of, and thus more vulnerable to, sexual health problems.

Evidence from surveys with young people on sex and relationships education suggests that they often lack opportunities to think about and discuss their own sexuality in a positive and safe environment. Such opportunities are vital to enable them to make informed judgements about the information they get from other sources. This is especially important in an era when access to pornography via the internet now appears to be one of the main sources young people use to learn about sexual behaviour. There is growing evidence that internet pornography is influencing and distorting young people's understanding of what is desirable, and/or appropriate, sexual behaviour in ways that increase risks to their sexual and psychological health and well-being (Papadopoulos, 2011).

So what is healthy sexual development? In Chapter 2, we saw that, in purely biological terms, adolescence is primarily about developing the physiological capacity to reproduce. This is reflected in the major hormonally driven physiological changes which occur during this life stage. We also saw that this process is highly variable in its timing and pace, reflecting the influence of both intrinsic factors, such as genetics, and extrinsic factors, such as nutrition. Physiological development is only part of the story, however. Psychological and cultural factors play a more significant role in the development of 'sexuality', as defined above, and add layers of complexity to our understanding of what healthy sexual development is. We must, for example, recognize the way that the cultural diversity of the UK will influence the ways sexual development will be responded to, experienced and interpreted in different communities. Gender, marital status, social class, place of residence, age, ethnicity, sexual orientation, level and type of sexual experience (whether voluntary or involuntary), motivations for sexual activity (affection, status, peer/partner pressure) and health status, are all among the diverse influences that shape the development of sexuality in individuals and across populations. And to complicate things even further, the notion of what is 'sexually healthy' may vary from generation to generation. Indeed, the idea of what constitutes sexual health can change even within the same individual. What may have been considered 'healthy' at age 15 may not be considered so at age 45.

The notion of a healthy sexuality is not, therefore, static and judgement-free. Sexual development occurs over a lifetime and is complex and difficult to make generalizations about. We do know, however, that the attainment of adult sexual health is closely linked to experiences during adolescence. And we also know that the smoothness of the transition from childhood to adolescence is influenced by the experiences of childhood. Adolescence is, then, the pivotal period of transition to adulthood and lays the foundations for sexual health in later life (Ford, 2005).

The way in which individuals experience puberty and awareness of their own developing sexual identity may vary considerably, but for most young people certain influences will be crucial. In particular:

- The response and reactions of parents and other key adults in their lives.

- The level of support they receive at school, and particularly the quality of Sex and Relationships Education (SRE).

- The all-important peer group around the young person.

- And, increasingly, the role of the media and marketing industries – especially the music, fashion and beauty industries, other media phenomena such as so-called reality TV, and the growing influence of internet pornography.

At a psychological level sexuality is very much about our sense of identity – who we feel we are, what we feel about ourselves and others, what we value, and what we desire. It is about understanding and experiencing what it means to become a man or woman, and what happens if one does not fit into the generally accepted ideas, or social stereotypes, of what those categories imply.

Sexuality also includes managing the different dimensions of relationships, whether they are sexual or not, including the degree of control and agency we have; whether sexual activities involve violence and coercion; and also, critically, our sense of self-worth and self-esteem, and the links between pleasure and desire.

Being sexual is also linked to the social, economic and educational opportunities available to us, and the impact of growing up in different cultures and social classes. All influence our decisions about when, where and how to be sexually active – or not – and how we respond to and interpret information about sexuality and sexual health. In modern, consumerist societies young people are often bombarded with images of idealized and sexualized bodies through targeted advertising, fashion, music and pornography – images that are often designed to promote feelings of inadequacy. The issue of how we promote 'healthy' responses and attitudes towards sexual development in young people is one that quality Sex and Relationships Education in schools and colleges should be addressing, alongside a more responsible approach from the media and other industries. We will look at these issues further below, but first, what are the key sexual health issues facing young people in the UK?

The key sexual health issues for young people

The past 20 years have seen an, at times, almost frenzied media response to the portrayal of young people and the key sexual health issues they face; so much so that one would be forgiven for believing that it is the norm for most teenagers to be sexually active, have multiple partners, contract multiple STIs and become parents before their sixteenth birthday – none of which is actually supported by evidence. We need, therefore, to look beyond the media headlines to gain a clear picture of what the real sexual health issues are for young people.

When students and professionals working with children and young people are asked to discuss what they believe to be the key issues the most popular response is undoubtedly teenage pregnancy, followed closely by STIs. Whilst these are key indicators of the state of young people's sexual health and well-being, young people themselves often highlight other issues that also need our consideration. We will consider the following areas:

- Sexual vulnerability – who is a sexually vulnerable young person, and what are the risk factors?

- The sexualization of young people

- Homophobia

- Teenage pregnancy
- Sexually Transmitted Infections

Who is a sexually vulnerable young person?

By their very nature, all young people could be considered sexually vulnerable, but certain factors place some young people at greater risk than most. Young people are known to be at greater risk of experiencing sexual health issues if they fit within one or more of the categories listed below:

• Live in an area of social deprivation	• Domestic violence
• Low education attainment	• Asylum seekers & refugees
• Poor school attendance – NEETs	• Teenage parents
• Living in or leaving Care	• Have been previously sexually abused
• Young offenders	• Homeless
• Poor mental health & learning disabilities	• Being under 13 and sexually active
• Substance misuse	• Unsure of sexuality

Young people who are sexually vulnerable often tend to have low self-esteem, low aspirations and low expectations. A sexually vulnerable young person is more likely to have a higher than average number of sexual partners, and thus be more at risk of contracting STIs. They are also the young people least likely to access sexual health services, often because they lack the confidence or means to get to these services, or because they are more likely to have a lack of confidence and trust in the 'helping' professions. Young people in this position have higher rates of unplanned pregnancies, without adequate support or means of accessing that support. And these factors often mean that there is a greater risk to psychological well-being too (DH & DCSF, 2010).

Surveys over the last decade have indicated that unwanted sex is not uncommon in young people's relationships. In 2008 the WAFE/Bliss survey reported that 'a quarter of all 14 year old girls have been coerced into sexual acts' (WAFE/Bliss 2008). A BBC online survey in 2006, in which 19,250 young people aged between 16 and 24 years old took part, showed that a third had had sex for the first time before the age of 16, and a quarter of those said that they had felt under pressure when having sex for the first time. A third had also drunk alcohol before having first-time sex, and a quarter had used no contraception (BBC Radio 1 Bare All youth sex survey, 2006). Evidence suggests that contraception is less likely to be used when sex is coerced. This suggests that there are close links between teenage pregnancy rates and sexual activity taking place under various levels of coercion. It is particularly poignant that one in five young men, and nearly half of young women aged between 16 and 24, said that they wished they had waited longer to start having sex (FPA 2007). More disturbingly, over a third of all rapes recorded by the police are committed against children and young people under 16 years of age (NSPCC, 2010).

This all suggests that it is more important than ever that Sex and Relationships Education is provided as part of the core curriculum available to young people. It is particularly important that young people are given the opportunity to develop communication, decision-making and negotiation skills, including how to resist pressure in relationships. Young people need to have the opportunity to identify what they feel comfortable with in a relationship, how to manage their own safety and personal boundaries, and the opportunity to rehearse these skills and strategies in a safe and supportive learning environment. This is what Holland et al. (1998) refer to as 'intellectual' empowerment – the ability to act on their knowledge and understanding.

Critically, young people and their families also need to know that when they do report sexual abuse, unwanted sexual attention or grooming activities to the police, social services or other professions and agencies, their report will be responded to and acted upon. Recent major scandals concerning widespread sexual abuse of young women in a number of UK cities have highlighted the importance of this. In those cases it appears that the young women in question were either not believed, or were effectively 'written off' because of a troubled personal or family history. As a result the vulnerability of those young women was compounded by the negative response of the very agencies that were supposed to protect them. In these cases the authorities, agencies and professions designed to protect vulnerable young people failed to do so, and it is imperative that the lessons of how and why that happened are learned so those problems are not repeated. It is also important to note that it was not the sexual attitudes and behaviours of the young people involved that was the problem in these cases, but those of many of the adults around them, which links us into the next issue – the growing sexualization of young people in the UK.

The sexualization of young people

Over the last decade there has been a growing sense that there has been a shift that is making our culture more 'pornified' or 'sexualized'; however, there continues to be much debate about what has changed, why it has changed and how these changes should be understood. We must begin with the question: 'what do we mean by sexualization?' What is clear from the media coverage of the subject is that we are not even sure that we are talking about the same thing when we use the term 'sexualization'.

'Sexualization' of young people means to 'make sexual in character or quality', and sexualized images suggest 'sexual availability to the exclusion of other personal characteristics and qualities', and in ways that are inappropriate, obscene, and harmful to children and young people (Collins English Dictionary, 2013). Definitions can be helpful but for the time being it is still not clear whether those participating in the debate are clear on the phenomenon they are talking about. In recent years the issue of the 'sexualization' of young people has attracted increasing amounts of attention from parents, politicians, children's rights campaigners, academics and researchers, and the popular press. Although there are diverse agendas and motives surrounding this emotive debate, there is widespread agreement that the world that young people now grow up in is far more sexualized – including sexually explicit music lyrics, sexually charged music videos and sexualized clothing marketed to parents and so-called tweenagers (pre-teen girls mainly) – than that experienced by previous generations. This concern has led to a response from the highest levels of government. Dr Linda Papadopoulos was commissioned by the Home Office to conduct an independent review of the impact of the sexualization of young girls on violence against women. The intention of the review was to contribute to a wider debate about the risk to children's developmental well-being through the sexualization process. She reviewed research on the 'objectification' of girls and the 'hyper-masculinization' of boys, and how they interact to reinforce each other (Papadopoulos, 2011).

The key findings of this review were:

- The increasingly widespread sexualization of children and young people in music, fashion and computer games

- The increasing availability of, exposure to, and extreme nature of, pornography

- The pervasive and insidious impact of unreal and manipulated body images

- Young people's apparent lack of awareness of gender equality issues

Papadopoulos proposed that government become more proactive in pressurizing and regulating advertisers, retailers, broadcasters, and the gaming and IT industries to act responsibly. She also recommended that the government make it easier for parents and young people to report and complain about inappropriate advertising and marketing, and to have a greater voice in framing the debate about sexualization.

The Papadopoulos Review was followed up in 2011 by *Letting Children be Children*, another government-commissioned report, this time undertaken by Reg Bailey, chief executive of the Mothers' Union, focusing on the commercialization and sexualization of childhood (Department of Education, 2011). The Bailey Review aimed to assess the nature and extent to which children and young people are pressurized into 'growing up too quickly'. Bailey called for businesses, regulators and the Government to play their part and protect children from the increasingly sexualized 'wallpaper' that surrounds them (Bailey, 2011, pp. 17, 18). Prime Minister David Cameron gave his strong support to the proposals to 'shield children from sexualised imagery across the media and tackle the commercialisation of childhood', but has been reluctant to back change through government regulation, preferring an emphasis on voluntary 'social responsibility'.

The increased accessibility to young people of pornography via the internet is an area of major concern, particularly with the spread of internet access via smart phones. The Office of the Children's Commissioner published the report *Basically Porn is Everywhere* (2013) calling for urgent action to develop young people's resilience to pornography. The report highlighted evidence that pornography influences many young people's attitudes towards their own relationships and sexuality, and also found links to risky behaviour, such as having sex at a younger age, and a correlation between holding violent attitudes and accessing media containing sexual violence (Horvath et al., 2013). The suggestion here is that early exposure to pornography can lead to premature sexual activity; however, evidence is largely anecdotal and more empirical research needs to be carried out before such claims can be made. There is, however, increasing evidence of a connection between exposure to media images and poor body image, self-harming and eating disorders.

We can be in no doubt that there is widespread and growing concern about 'sexualization' and this can be seen in public and policy reports as well as in the growing array of popular books on the subject. From the sensationalist perspective of Sue Palmer's 'Toxic Childhood', to the 2010 'Review of the Sexualisation of Young People' by Linda Papadopoulos, to the Bailey Report, *Letting Children Be Children* (2011), there appears to be an assumption that there is overwhelming evidence that children and young people, and particularly girls, are 'directly sexualized' through their exposure to the media. However, whilst there is no shortage of anecdotal and sensationalist media coverage of the subject there is, in fact, a distinct shortage of rigorous research on what many consider to be **the** emotive issue of the early twenty-first century. (Gill cited in *Premature Sexualisation: the risks – Outcomes of the NSPCC expert seminars series.* [2011, pp. 4, 5]). Practitioners working with children and young people should be aware that academics such as Emma Renold, Jessica Ringrose and E. Danielle Egan (2015) are critical of some of the assumptions made by Palmer, Papadopoulos and Bailey. Renold et al. bring together empirical studies and discourse that suggest that in order to understand what is happening now we need to acknowledge the historical context and the conceptualization of childhood that has taken place. We need to understand how the ideas about childhood sexuality have developed. There have been ongoing debates throughout the nineteenth and twentieth centuries regarding the influence of 'sexually salacious sources', such as comic strips, television and music, upon children and young people, and that this becomes more apparent in times of upheaval, be it during times of economic depression or social conflict (Renold et al., 2015, p. 3). Renold et al. welcome the long overdue attention being given to the significance and representation of sexuality and how this might be shaping children's and young people's sexual cultures, but in doing so they call for a more detailed examination of what we mean by the concept of 'sexualization' (Renold et al., 2015).

The debate on the 'sexualization of children' continues but the challenge for those working with and supporting young people is how to respond to the issue of the growing presence of pornography in society without falling foul of accusations of censorship and the curtailing of freedoms? One strategy being adopted in schools and colleges with more robust Sex and Relationships Education programmes is to give young people the opportunity to discuss sensitive issues such as pornography and consent within the comparatively safe learning environment of the classroom. What is becoming increasingly apparent is that any work with young people around their sexual behaviour and sexual health has to acknowledge and confront the 'sexualized' world that they live in and to include strategies that challenge the confusing messages young people receive (Brook, PSHE Association and Sex Education Forum, 2014, pp. 10, 11).

Homophobia

The tragic deaths of Damilola Taylor, Laura Rhodes and Jody Dobrowski may appear to have nothing in common to many people, but those with an understanding of the culture of homophobic bullying that exists in schools are able to see the link very clearly. These were three young people for whom sexuality, or their perceived sexuality, was such an issue in their lives that it played a role in their deaths. These tragedies, together with pressure from campaign groups such as Stonewall, have put pressure on the government and schools to address the issue of homophobia.

There is little official research on this subject, but in recent years a number of independent studies have presented a damning picture of what it is like to be young and gay, or perceived by others to be gay. A study published in 2006, for example, based on a survey with young people in Calderdale and Kirklees, found that 70 per cent of young gay people had had suicidal thoughts, and that

61 per cent had actually attempted suicide, whilst 87 per cent had self-harmed. In 2006, Stonewall published findings from a survey of young people which found that less than a quarter of young gay people have been told that homophobic bullying is wrong in their school. In schools that have given a clear message that homophobic bullying is wrong young gay people are 60 per cent less likely to have been bullied.

Stonewall offer training aimed at giving education professionals an increased understanding of homophobic bullying, and provide a range of practical and effective strategies to challenge it (www.stonewall.org.uk). Every secondary school in the country received a training pack and were also given opportunities to access training and support to help them feel confident in tackling the issues. This marked an important step towards tackling the homophobic bullying that damages the lives of so many young people. Despite this progress, however, training packs and resources are not enough if teachers themselves and the schools as institutions are not prepared, or feel supported, to challenge homophobia in the first place.

'Schools should be discussing gay issues in assemblies and introducing novels for English classes with LGBT themes,' says Sue Sanders, co-chair of School's Out, which campaigns against homophobia in education. She added, 'Many schools study the work of Jackie Kay in English [Literature] and, while they will almost certainly talk about race, they rarely mention her sexuality' (*The Guardian*, 31 July 2006).

In 2012, Stonewall published its 'School Report', indicating that there is still a long way to go before homophobia in schools is truly addressed and challenged. The report concluded:

- Homophobic bullying continues to be widespread in Britain's schools. More than half (55 per cent) of lesbian, gay and bisexual pupils have experienced direct bullying;

- The use of homophobic language is endemic. Almost all (99 per cent) gay young people hear the phrases 'that's so gay' or 'you're so gay' in school and 96 per cent of gay pupils hear homophobic language such as 'poof' or 'lezza';

- Three in five gay pupils who experience homophobic bullying say that teachers who witness the bullying never intervene;

- Only half of gay pupils report that their schools say homophobic bullying is wrong. Even fewer faith schools (37 per cent) do;

- Homophobic bullying has a profoundly damaging impact on young people's school experience. One in three (32 per cent) gay pupils experiencing bullying change their future educational plans because of it, and three in five say it impacts directly on their school work;

- Gay people who are bullied are at a higher risk of suicide, self-harm and depression. Two in five (41 per cent) have attempted or thought about taking their own life directly because of bullying and the same number say that they deliberately self-harm directly because of bullying.

There has been some progress, however. Local authorities and other agencies are beginning to respond to the issue. For example, since 2006:

- The rate of homophobic bullying of lesbian, gay and bisexual young people has decreased from 65 per cent to 55 per cent;
- Twice as many gay pupils report that their schools say homophobic bullying is wrong – 50 per cent, up from 25 per cent in 2007;
- The number of gay pupils who still feel unable to speak out when they are bullied, whilst still too high, has fallen from 58 per cent to 37 per cent.

(School Report, 2012, Stonewall)

Efforts have been made then, but local authorities, the new academy schools and youth organizations such as the Scouts and Guides cannot afford to be complacent. Encouragingly, the recent Ofsted framework (2012), with its key judgement area on 'Behaviour and Safety' and its emphasis on the school's duty to promote the 'Spiritual, Moral, Social and Cultural' development of pupils, informs schools that inspectors will be *'exploring the school's actions to prevent homophobic bullying'*.

Attitudes and behaviours are difficult to shift, as Alan Wardle, the then Director for Parliamentary Affairs for Stonewall, and now Head of Corporate Affairs at the NSPCC, made clear back in 2007 when he said:

> Societal, cultural and attitude change is something that takes a long time. We're in it for the long haul.

We still have a long way to go to eliminate homophobic bullying from schools. It should be a basic expectation that all pupils in our schools should be able to complete their studies without experiencing the problem of bullying, but it remains the case that many young people are denied the opportunity to achieve their full academic potential because of homophobic bullying, exclusion and harassment.

Teenage parenthood

Teenage parenthood has been seen as a significant public health and social problem by successive British governments in recent decades. And the UK is not alone. By the late 1990s, 8 of the 28 OECD countries were engaged in interventions aimed at reducing teenage conceptions (UNICEF, 2001). Policy makers and the media have claimed that teenage parenthood ruins lives, both of the young parents and their children, and even threatens to destroy the very social and moral fabric of society (DH & DCSF, 2010).

Recent research suggests that this is not such a clear-cut issue, however. Not only is the perception that teenage pregnancy has spiralled out of control since the late twentieth century incorrect, but evidence also suggests that early parenthood is not necessarily the disaster it is made out to be. Recent research has actually indicated that teenage fertility rates are considerably lower today than they were in the 1960s, and that it is the socioeconomic background of the mother, the availability and quality of support networks and services that are the key issues. It also appears that becoming a teenage parent can sometimes improve the lives of young parents (Duncan, 2010; Arai, 2009).

Duncan et al. (2010) take the argument further, asserting that there is a media-perpetuated myth of a 'teenage pregnancy epidemic', generating a negative public consensus around teenage pregnancy. They argue that this consensus is based on the ill-founded assumption that teenage pregnancy is increasing rapidly, and that this increase is particularly apparent in younger teenagers. The assumption created, they argue, is that all teenage pregnancies are unplanned and unwanted, and that teenage mothers are inevitably single mothers without the benefits of stable relationships with the babies' fathers. Research data appear to tell a different story. Far from witnessing a rapid increase in teenage parenthood, we have actually seen a substantial decline in both birth rates and absolute numbers of births to teenagers since the 1960s and early 1970s (see Table 7.1, adapted from Duncan et al., 2008, p. 10).

Table 7.1 Live births and birth rates for women under 20, 1951–2008 adapted from table 1, Duncan et al. (2008, p. 10)

Year	No of live births	Birth rate per 1000 women aged 15–19
1951	29,111	21.3
1961	37,938	27.3
1971	82,641	50.6
1981	60,800	30.9
1991	52,396	33.1
2001	44,189	28.0
2007	44,805	26.0

These data only show 'live births' of children born to mothers under 20, and do not give us an indication of how many conceptions ended in terminations during the same period. We know, however, that prior to the 1967 Abortion Act, teenagers not prepared to go through with 'shotgun marriages' often dealt with unplanned or unwanted pregnancies by illegal abortion or adoption. More recent data on teenage pregnancy and birth rates suggest that more pregnant teenagers opt for giving birth rather than termination even though this can now be done both legally and safely (Smith, 1993). Also, there are very few teenage mothers – only 6 per cent in 2006 – accounting for only 0.9 per cent of all births in Britain by 2007. Overall, teenage birth rates are now at the same levels as they were in the 1950s. The crucial difference is that in the 1950s and 1960s the majority of teenage parents were married to partners who were earning a wage sufficient to support them (Duncan et al., 2008).

Debates around the causes and consequences of teenage parenthood, and ways of dealing with it, have evolved according to shifts in the political climate. Conservative governments in the 1980s and 1990s adopted a predominantly punitive approach, demonizing young single mothers. In contrast, the New Labour governments between 1997 and 2010 linked teenage pregnancy to social exclusion rather than personal morality, and aimed, through its Teenage Pregnancy Strategy (TPS), to reduce teenage pregnancy through better sex education, access to sexual health services, raising the aspirations of young people and supporting young mothers' participation in education and employment. The New Labour approach still held, however, to the mantra that teenage pregnancy was a social problem. Despite criticisms of the TPS, it undoubtedly brought with it unprecedented resources, both to the prevention of unwanted teenage pregnancies and support given to young parents. By 2012 teenage pregnancy rates had fallen to the lowest since 1969.

The election of the Coalition government in May 2010, with its 'austerity' programme and public spending cuts, continued with more vigour since the election of the Conservative government in 2015, has meant that the funding around support and services for both the prevention of teenage pregnancy and support for young parents has been substantially reduced. Despite debates amongst academics and in the media over whether the New Labour approach was correct or not, the data tell an interesting story. Undeniably, the pulling together of resources, agencies, support services, health, education, employment and housing had all begun to have an impact on teenage pregnancy rates in the UK, and it will be interesting to see how the change in the economic and political climate, alongside continuing cuts in support services, are reflected in future teenage pregnancy rates.

Young people and STIs

One of the main differences in the health issues facing young people in the UK now compared with 50 years ago is the virtual eradication – temporarily at least – of infectious disease as a major health risk. One exception stands out, however – STIs. A report published in 2010 from the Health Protection Agency indicates a worrying rise in STIs in those aged under 25 years. Sexual health clinics reported 482,700 new cases in 2009, a rise of 12,000 on the previous year, with two thirds of the increase presenting in young women aged 15–24. Of particular concern is the rise in the rate of Chlamydia infection. But there are also worrying upwards trends too in other STIs, including Gonorrhoea, Syphilis, Genital Warts and HIV (HPA, 2009).

Human Immunodeficiency Virus (HIV) is the STI that makes most headlines around the world because of its links to the ultimately fatal condition AIDS, where the body succumbs to normally relatively harmless infections, such as Herpes, as the person's immune system becomes increasingly compromised. HIV can be transmitted in a number of ways, including needle sharing among drug users. But transmission by either anal or vaginal intercourse is by far the main cause of the spread of infection – 95 per cent in the UK in 2011 for instance. There remains no cure for HIV, although new antiretroviral drug treatments mean that people can now live much longer before developing AIDS. Undoubtedly, the most effective strategy preventing the spread of HIV infection is the use of condoms – and this is true of most STIs (NHS Choices Website, 2014).

The full health impact of most untreated STIs tends to be delayed – sometimes by many years, or even decades. After an initial show of discomforting symptoms, such as a burning sensation during urination with Gonorrhoea, or a small sore in the genital area with Syphilis, for example, all goes quiet. In both these infections serious effects will emerge in later life, however. Gonorrhoea infection can lead to infertility, or Pelvic Inflammatory Disease in women. Whilst the bacteria that causes Syphilis will, if untreated, go on to cause devastating, and ultimately fatal, nerve and neurological damage in later life. Thankfully, the devastating symptoms of so-called tertiary (3rd stage) Syphilis are now rare in the UK, as the infection is usually spotted much earlier (NHS Choices Website, 2014).

The STI of most concern in relation to young people in the UK is Chlamydia. In 2012 over 200,000 people tested positive for Chlamydia in England, 64 per cent of whom were under 25. An insidious characteristic of Chlamydia is that it often produces no noticeable symptoms. Hence, one of the main strategies being used is to encourage people under 25 to undergo free voluntary screening as part of the National Chlamydia Screening Programme (NCSP), which can be accessed in Colleges, Universities, pharmacies, GU Clinics and GP surgeries. Untreated Chlamydia can lead to infertility and/or Pelvic Inflammatory Disease in later life (NHS Choices Website, 2014).

Unlike HIV infection, bacterial STIs, such as Chlamydia, Gonorrhoea and Syphilis, can all be cured using antibiotics. But the main approach used to counter their spread is preventative education encouraging the use of condoms. The data on STIs within the 15 to 25 age group suggest that, whilst we have seen a relatively successful outcome in the campaign to bring down teenage pregnancies, the message about safe sex and wider sexual health is not getting through to the extent needed to bring down STI infection rates. The Department of Health's 'A framework for Sexual Health Improvement in England' (2013) has made clear its ambition to build knowledge and resilience, and improve sexual health outcomes for young people. The report recognizes that more needs to be done, however, to ensure messages regarding 'safe sex' are understood and applied by sexually active young people. This leads us on to look at strategies used to try to improve the sexual health of young people.

The campaign for quality Sex and Relationships Education (SRE)

The main overall strategy for promoting sexual health in young people has been the delivery of Sex and Relationships Education in schools. During the era of the New Labour governments a campaign was launched to make Personal, Social, Health and Economic education (PSHE education) a statutory subject, and also a move to make Sex and Relationships Education (SRE) a compulsory component of the national curriculum. Bodies such as the Sex Education Forum and the PSHE Association were joined by colleagues from a range of organizations and backgrounds, such as the Family Planning Association (FPA) and local Teenage Pregnancy Partnership Boards, in calling for SRE to be a statutory subject for all pupils. A National PSHE Continuous Professional Development (CPD) Programme was launched with funding to train a teacher and/or a community nurse in every school to achieve accreditation against new national standards for the teaching of PSHE education (including SRE). In 2002, the Office for Standards in Education (Ofsted) published a report in response to the SEU's *Teenage Pregnancy Report* that it should carry out a survey on the quality of Sex and Relationships Education. The key findings of the report were:

- Whilst schools adequately covered the factual aspects of human reproduction, teaching about parenthood, relationships and the prevention of infection was of poor quality.

- The DfES (2000) guidance on SRE had a positive effect on SRE provision in both primary and secondary schools, but many schools had still not reviewed their policies, and monitoring and evaluation of SRE was inadequate. SRE policies were poor in one in ten schools.

- In secondary schools teaching about sexual health and the law in relation to sex was poor in one in five lessons, although teaching about contraception was good, particularly at KS 4.

- Education about parenthood did not feature in all secondary schools programmes. Boys reported that not much in their SRE lessons was relevant to them.

Whilst the report agreed that reducing the incidence of teenage pregnancy was very important, it recognized also that it was not the only purpose of SRE. The report highlighted other important factors to be considered, including to:

- Broaden the definitions of achievement in SRE to include development of pupils' values, attitudes and personal skills, making clear what pupils should learn by the end of each key stage.

- Provide further advice on content and methods for teaching about parenthood and sexuality for teachers and within this a recommendation that schools should develop expert teams of teachers to deliver all aspects of PSHE education including SRE – linked to the government target to have accredited PSHE teachers/health professionals in every secondary school.

- Focus more attention within the secondary curriculum to cover the prevention of STIs including HIV/AIDS and Chlamydia.

- Provide more advice and support for parents, especially fathers.

- Encourage LEAs and Health Authorities to consider how pupils can have better access to individual advice from specialists both at school and outside of school.

- Ensure values and codes of behaviour were consistently adhered to, e.g. homophobic attitudes are challenged along with derogatory comments and unacceptable language.

(OFSTED, 2002)

The report was broadly welcomed by campaigners for statutory SRE and the following decade saw an unprecedented focus of resources and expertise to improve the quality of both sex education and sexual health support for young people. In 2008, a government review of SRE was undertaken and recommended that PSHE be made part of the statutory curriculum for schools and that all children receive at least one year of SRE (Children, Schools and Families Bill, Session 2009–2010). To the dismay of the campaigners, however, these elements of the Bill were lost in the parliamentary 'wash up' on the dissolution of Parliament for the general election of May 2010.

In 2011 the Coalition government launched its own review of PSHE education, and in 2013 Education Minister Michael Gove announced the government's review of the entire National Curriculum and, as many had anticipated,

PSHE was to remain non-statutory. Campaigners drew some comfort, however, from the statement within the curriculum announcement that:

> All schools **should** make provision for personal, social, health and economic education (PSHE), drawing on good practice. (National Curriculum, Section 2.3, 2013)

In 2015 the government issued a House of Commons briefing notice that stated:

> All maintained secondary schools must provide sex and relationship education as part of the basic curriculum, and must meet the requirements of National Curriculum Science. (House of Commons Briefing Paper 16 July 2015, number 06103: 4)

In 2014, the PSHE Association, Brook and Sex Education Forum, funded by the Department of Education, published supplementary guidance to the 2000 Sex and Relationship Guidance (DfEE, 2000). This gives guidance on addressing issues such as 'consent', 'sexualization' and the 'impact of pornography'. These developments have all been welcomed by campaigners for quality SRE in schools. The message from the Department of Education is still often ambiguous, however, about what is actually statutory and what remains guidance. The campaign to make PSHE and SRE compulsory subjects in schools continues.

Professionals working around PSHE education and in the delivery of Sex and Relationships Education know that schools are currently faced with an increasingly squeezed curriculum which appears to be judged solely on results in English and Maths. It will mainly be down, therefore, to the enthusiasm and commitment of individual teachers and professionals to ensure that children and young people really do get access to a broad and relevant curriculum which truly equips them for the challenges of twenty-first-century life.

What does quality SRE look like?

Evidence from bodies such as the PSHE Association and the Sex Education Forum, and on evidence-based practice such as that evaluated by Kirby (2002 and 2009), suggests that the most effective sexual health promotion with young people calls for the focus to be on the following key factors:

- Know and understand the needs of your target group
- Involve the experts in planning and delivery
- Focus on specific types of behaviour, e.g. abstaining from sex, using condoms; giving clear messages about types of behaviour, etc.
- Create a safe learning environment and use effective evidence-based teaching and learning strategies

- Messages about healthy relationships need to start early and to be part of the primary curriculum. The earlier the better!

- SRE should be part of a planned and progressive curriculum from nursery to Year 11

- SRE needs to be relevant and appropriate to children and young people – addressing some of the more sensitive and controversial issues such as body image, the media and the impact of pornography on young people

- SRE needs to be delivered in partnership with children, young people, parents/carers, teachers and health professionals. Young people need to be involved in the designing, planning, implementation and evaluation of the SRE curriculum

- Deliverers of SRE need to be appropriately trained

- SRE and sexual health messages need to be delivered alongside provision of advice and access to services

- SRE and messages about sexual health need to concentrate on skills, attitudes and behaviours and not just knowledge. Young people need to be able to apply their knowledge, using skills such as negotiation and reasoning to ensure the best outcomes for themselves.

The status of SRE remains, all too often, a 'political football' kicked at regular intervals between various political parties. The debate is often framed as 'parental rights and responsibilities' versus 'children and young people's entitlement to effective SRE'. Should under 16 year olds have access to sexual health advice and contraception without parental knowledge or consent? The Gillick Case, 1983, brought the dilemma of giving under 16s contraceptive advice to the public attention. Victoria Gillick wrote to her local area health authority seeking an assurance that no contraceptive advice or treatment would be given to her daughters without her knowledge and consent. In 1983 this ended up in the High Court, where Mrs Gillick's claim that it was unlawful for any NHS worker to give advice to her daughter without parental consent was dismissed. However, in December 1984 the Appeal Court overturned this ruling, and Mrs Gillick's declaration was granted with immediate effect. The issue rested on the importance of parental consent and, except for advice in an 'emergency' or 'with leave of the Court', healthcare professionals were deemed to be acting illegally if they provided contraceptive advice or treatment to a girl under 16 without the consent of her parents. The immediate consequence of this ruling was a huge drop in the number of under 16s attending family planning clinics. An appeal to the House of Lords in October 1985 led to a new ruling that the guidance given to doctors by the Department of Health and

Social Services was not unlawful. Following this decision, the guidance was reinstated immediately, although a full review was announced to take account of the Law Lords' judgments and the wide range of views expressed on the issue. The debate surrounding parental rights and responsibilities versus children and young people's rights continues to influence the nature of the debate around Sex and Relationships Education. Such a confrontational approach seems more to hinder, rather than help, efforts to make SRE a statutory requirement of all schools, and to ensure young people are empowered with the knowledge and skills they need to negotiate this complex area of life. The preferred approach of professional bodies such as the PSHE Association and the Sex Education Forum is for schools to work in partnership with parents and the community to ensure that their children have access to relevant and age appropriate Sex and Relationships Education (Brook, PSHE Association and Sex Education Forum, 2014).

Conclusions

Whilst the issues surrounding the sexual health and well-being of young people are very real, and likely to continue as a high-priority area of concern, to some extent issues such as 'teenage pregnancy' seem to have fallen – temporarily, we suspect – off the policy agenda and disappeared from the headlines of the tabloid press. Calls to make SRE a statutory requirement are still being made, and teenage pregnancy continues to be mentioned as a significant problem, despite indications that rates are falling. But whilst the latest figures (ONS, 2015), based on data collected in 2013, show that England's teenage pregnancy rates are falling, the rates of teen pregnancies in England remain the highest in Western Europe. Despite the downward trend, many working in the field suggest that the reduction is largely due to the success of the 10-year Teenage Pregnancy Strategy (TPS), which ended in 2010 (FPA spokesperson cited in *The Guardian*, 15 July 2015). Perhaps the TPS has lost its impetus? Perhaps this is due to a growing realization that the ambitious teenage pregnancy targets of the New Labour government made in 1999 are unlikely to be met in coming years and other high profile 'youth issues' have pushed teenage pregnancy out of the limelight. Downs' (1972) work on the 'issue-attention' cycle of social problems describes how social issues often go through cycles of public attention. The 'moral panic' that once surrounded youth sexuality and teenage parenthood is now being applied more to obesity, with similar language being adopted such as 'obesity hot spots' and 'obesity epidemic'. However, when teenage pregnancy or the sexual behaviour of young people is mentioned, it too often continues to be reported in a sensational and alarmist way.

When it comes to the sexual well-being of young people society's response always seems to be muddied by the conflicting ways in which sexual well-being is understood. Different commentators and stakeholders are all influenced by personal values, religion, political ideology, socioeconomic factors, culture, education and our own experiences. What we must remember is that whilst there are clearly young people who experience a turbulent and confusing adolescence, the majority of young people do not and most will go on to have good sexual health and happy and healthy relationships.

8

NUTRITION, HEALTH AND YOUNG PEOPLE

In this chapter we will explore issues relating to young people's nutrition, and their sometimes complex relationship with food and eating. In particular, we will explore issues related to eating disorders, such as anorexia nervosa and bulimia nervosa, and look at the issue of obesity. These are some of the most worrying, and widely discussed, health issues affecting young people today, and there is much debate over how we should respond as a society and the relative roles and responsibilities of parents, media, advertising, the food industry and government.

Food and nutrition is, of course, basic to good health. Human beings need good nutrition to function well. During the developmental periods of childhood and adolescence good nutrition is critical to building healthy bodies and minds, and poor nutrition at this time can have serious long-term health consequences that play out over the rest of the lifespan. This is also the period of life in which many health-related behaviours – including eating habits – become established and entrenched. Food is also intrinsically linked to our emotional health and well-being. Pretty et al. (2009) identify the importance of establishing 'healthy pathways' during childhood, showing that, although patterns of eating and exercise are by no means unchangeable in later life, the healthiest option is to establish optimum patterns early on.

Besides the more extreme eating disorders, however, there is also a more general concern about young people's nutrition. The eating habits of the twenty-first century are very different to those of previous generations. Changes in the way we cook, preserve and access foods have had a profound effect. The population of the UK as a whole are, for example, eating less fruit and vegetables than they were a decade ago. This trend has been further exacerbated by the current economic climate. What are the implications of these changes for young people?

The impact of poor nutrition

The National Diet and Nutrition Survey (2011) reports that there is cause for concern regarding the general nutritional standards of the food young people are consuming. In particular:

- The average consumption of saturated fat, sugar and salt is too high.

- The consumption of starchy carbohydrates and fibre is low.

- In 7 days more than half the young people surveyed had not eaten any citrus fruits, green leafy vegetables, eggs or raw tomatoes.

- One in ten teenagers have very low intakes of vitamin A, magnesium, zinc, potassium, iron and calcium.

The Survey also used diet diaries to collect information on young people's (aged 11–18 years) dietary habits. The results revealed low levels of daily intake of a variety of minerals such as iron, selenium and magnesium. Looking specifically at iron deficiency, for example, one of the most common nutritional deficiencies in the UK, up to 13 per cent of teenage boys and 27 per cent of girls were found to have low iron stores. This can have a negative impact on concentration and energy levels. Iron is also necessary for periods of rapid physical growth, such as the growth spurts that take place in and around puberty. Teenage girls need to take particular care as their iron stores can also be depleted by menstruation, raising the risk of anaemia.

Likewise, 25 per cent of teenagers have been found to have calcium levels below the recommended level, which can have serious implications for their future bone health. Bones continue to grow and strengthen until the age of 30 and the teenage years are very important for this development. Vitamin D, calcium and phosphorous are all vital in this process and depend on a healthy and varied diet. Low calcium levels in adolescence have been linked to osteoporosis in later life, particularly in women; a condition that causes bones to become brittle and break easily. And it is not just what, but also how and when we eat that matters. Skipping breakfast, for example, sends messages to our brains that appear to instruct our bodies to go into hibernation mode, meaning any calories that we do consume will be hoarded for later and stored as fat. Skipping breakfast can also result in mood swings, an inability to concentrate and increase feelings of hunger for the rest of the day. The UNICEF (2013) report on the well-being of children revealed that 40 per cent of children aged 11–18 report that they do not eat a daily breakfast – despite evidence that breakfast is the most important meal of the day (Pivak et al., 2012; Hoyland et al., 2009). Teachers, too, report that, as the current economic climate takes hold, more children are arriving at school having missed breakfast, with increasing numbers reporting that the last meal they had was the school lunch of the previous day. It is well established that well-nourished young people are much more receptive to teaching and learn better, alongside the other health benefits of a balanced and nutritious diet.

Physical activity and young people

Levels of physical activity play a critical role too, not only in maintaining a healthy weight, but also in achieving overall health and well-being (Department of Health, 2011a). The 'Health Behaviour in School Aged Children' surveys in England and Scotland (Department of Health, 2011b) show that the proportion of young people aged 11–15 who were meeting the recommended levels for physical activity were only 28 per cent of boys and 15 per cent of girls in England, and 19 per cent of boys and 11 per cent of girls in Scotland (AYPH, 2013).

Whilst in previous generations most young people attended schools within walking distance of their homes, increasing numbers are now 'ferried' to and from school either in their parents' car or by bus or train. Some 38 per cent of journeys to and from school by young people aged 11–16 are made on foot, with most of the rest making the journey by bus or car, whilst only 3 per cent make the journey by rail, and 3 per cent by bicycle (AYPH, 2013). Other evidence suggests that physical exercise is less common still among young people from vulnerable groups. Two significant examples of this are those who are disabled and those from poorer socioeconomic backgrounds (Department for Culture, Media and Sport, 2007).

Social influences and body image

The relationship of young people with food is also strongly influenced by social and cultural factors. The amount and range of food available to young people today is unprecedented, as is the amount of targeted marketing pressure on them from a hugely influential 'fast-food' industry. At the same time, young people are subject to intense marketing pressures from the fashion and music industries, and so-called celebrity culture, all of which tend to emphasize the importance of appearance – particularly the desirability of being thin and beautiful. At times it can seem as if young people are living in a kind of 'pressure-cooker' environment in which they are constantly encouraged to judge others, and themselves, by how they look above all else. One manifestation of this is a rise in the importance of body image, which is particularly implicated in the rise of eating disorders.

The term 'body image' refers to our understanding of, and feelings about, how our body looks, and how we believe it is perceived by others. It is the picture we hold in our minds about our own physical appearance which can be shaped by our mood, experiences and environment. We are all affected to some extent by these perceptions, but they are particularly powerful for young people. Being a transitional stage of physical and psychological development, adolescence is characterized by a rapid phase of physical growth and change, simultaneously becoming acutely aware of external influences and evaluations, both positive and negative. Puberty brings with it changing body shapes and often turbulent emotions that can leave young people susceptible to negative thoughts about their changing bodies.

The development of body image is complex, however, and it can be difficult to pinpoint the exact causes of negative body image. We know that it is closely related to self-esteem and self-evaluation, and findings from recent research, such as the APPG Inquiry into Body Image (2012), suggest that these are increasingly influenced by the pervasive media and marketing machine that bombards young people with images of thin and 'perfect' bodies. Surveys of young people over the last 15 years have revealed that a growing number are dissatisfied and unhappy with their bodies. For example:

- Almost one quarter of children aged 10–15 are unhappy about their appearance (ONS, 2012).

- Thirty-four per cent of adolescent boys and 49 per cent of girls have been on a diet to change their body shape or to lose weight (Centre for Appearance Research & Central YMCA, 2011). Forty-two per cent of girls and young women feel that the most negative part about being a female is the pressure to look attractive (Girl Guiding UK, Girls Attitude Survey, 2010).

- The Good Childhood Inquiry 2012 found that 10–15 per cent of young people reported that they were unhappy with their appearance (Children's Society, 2012).

- And 60 per cent of adults report that they feel ashamed of the way they look (Centre for Appearance Research, 2012).

Burrowes (2013) found that the groups most likely to suffer from body image issues include:

- Children and young people
- Gay men in comparison with heterosexual men
- Women in comparison with men – regardless of their ethnicity or age
- White and South East Asian adolescent girls are more at risk of body dissatisfaction than Afro-Caribbean girls – possibly due to different body ideals
- Individuals with low self-esteem and/or suffering from depression.

Why are young people so at risk?

Research in this area has focused mostly on adolescents, but in the last 10 years evidence has emerged to suggest that this is also an issue which is affecting younger children too (Hutchinson and Calland, 2011). Evidence submitted to the APPG (2012) suggests that children as young as 5 years old begin to recognize when they are 'different' from other people and to comprehend that they may be negatively judged because of this. Calland (2011) suggests that 5-year-old children are already aware that certain body types are more acceptable in society than others, and goes on to argue that it is not children that have changed but the social context in which increased emphasis is placed on appearance as the primary way to gain acceptance and be valued. The APPG report (2012) also argues that it is society that has changed rather than the cognitive abilities or sensitivities of young children. Their figures seem to speak for themselves:

- Over half of girls and a quarter of boys think their peers have body image problems.

- Between one third and half of young girls fear becoming fat and engage in dieting or binge eating.

- Girls as young as 5 years are worried about the way they look and their size.

- One in four 7-year-old girls have tried to lose weight at least once.

- One third of young boys aged 8–12 are dieting to lose weight.

The evidence points firmly at increased social and cultural pressure generated by the marketing strategies of 'the body-image' industries – fashion, beauty and music. Papadopoulos (2014) has argued, with particular reference to young women, that the rise of screen-based technologies means that they are now living in a primarily visual environment, where a disproportionate emphasis is placed on comparing themselves with others via social networking sites, and where appearance is valued above all other attributes, such as intelligence, resilience, determination and kindness. For young people in the process of developing their sense of self it is important to have opportunities to value themselves and others in as many different ways as possible. A healthy self-concept needs to draw on diverse sources to encourage self-development. The overbearing value placed on appearance appears to be overwhelming opportunities for young people to be exposed to other influences, however. Many will negotiate this body-image pressure without it turning into anything more sinister than a nagging sense of dissatisfaction. For an increasing amount of young people, however, it turns into a deeper source of unhappiness with themselves that can lead to something far more sinister and damaging.

Young people and eating disorders

Eating disorders affect around 1.6 million people in the UK, and most eating disorders tend to start in the mid-teens (NHS Choices, 2015). Understanding these complex and highly distressing conditions is therefore important for those working with young people. We will focus here on the two commonest eating disorders: anorexia nervosa and bulimia nervosa.

Anorexia nervosa

Anorexia nervosa is a disorder in which a person maintains a low weight as a result of a preoccupation with their own body weight, interpreted as a fear of fatness or an obsessive pursuit of thinness. Sufferers maintain their weight at levels that are at least 15 per cent below that regarded as normative. Diagnosis is often made at or just after puberty when the young person fails to make the weight gain and expected growth spurt normally associated with this physical change. Weight loss is achieved by avoiding 'fattening foods', sometimes alongside excessive exercising, and/or self-induced purging by vomiting or misuse of laxatives. This impairs the quality of nutritional intake and can lead to a widespread endocrine (hormone) disorder involving the hypothalamic-pituitary-gonadal axis which can halt the menstrual cycle in women, and in men manifests itself in a loss of sexual interest or potency. Although anorexia nervosa is rare in prepubertal children, where it does occur it can delay puberty and stunt physical development (Middleton, 2007).

The experience of the anorexia sufferer is often completely at odds with the concerns and assessment of the situation by those that love and care for them. The young person is often completely convinced that weight control is desirable and can strongly resist anyone who challenges this view. This is particularly the case when the individual is suffering from a poor sense of body image. In such circumstances weight loss is experienced as an achievement and something to be celebrated, and they will often deny that there is an issue (NICE, 2004).

A common experience appears to be that, initially, the condition starts with dieting behaviour that does not provoke any serious concern in those closest to the young person. Indeed some receive reinforcing compliments from friends and family members for losing weight. It is only when secondary features, such as social withdrawal and obsessive behaviours, develop that family and friends become concerned. These secondary features can have a damaging effect on the social and emotional development of a young person, compromising their future aspirations, employment opportunities, engagement in leisure and sporting activities, self-care and simple day-to-day living (Middleton, 2007).

A small proportion of young people will enter anorexia nervosa through a pattern of purging behaviour following a viral illness, such as glandular fever, which may have resulted in weight loss that then became positively valued. An even smaller number can enter anorexia nervosa as the result of a chronic illness, such as diabetes or Crohn's disease, where the individual has to be more aware of the types and frequency of food they are consuming, and, as a consequence, becomes acutely aware and controlling over the food they eat.

Normally, young people are persuaded to seek help by concerned family members, teachers or their GPs, who they may have consulted about the physical consequences they experience. Occasionally, the individual may appreciate the damaging effects of the disorder and seek help themselves. It is rare that a young person self-refers, however, and they are almost always brought to treatment by a family member (Bryant-Waugh et al., 1992 cited in NICE Guidance, 2004, p. 14). Diagnosis in young people is often complicated by the young person's own unwillingness to disclose his or her motives, symptoms and behaviours. It is usually their family or a concerned school teacher that makes the first contact with health professionals, expressing concerns over behaviours related to weight loss, such as:

- skipping meals

- hiding food

- adopting a restrictive diet

- changes in mood

- changes in sleep patterns

- increased physical activity or the adoption of gruelling exercise regimes.

When questioned, young people suffering from anorexia nervosa tend to display an exaggerated fear of gaining weight or becoming fat, despite being underweight, together with an inability to self-evaluate their body weight or body shape, and an obsessive preoccupation with their shape and weight-related matters. Not all of these features may be present, however, and the young person will often be quick to deny the seriousness of the weight loss. Those working with young people need to be skilled in engaging with them if they are to establish a climate of trust that enables them to discuss their fears about weight gain, eating and excessive exercising. Significant signs that should alert health professionals to the possibility of anorexia nervosa include:

- Physical features of starvation – such as skeletal appearance, abundance of downy-type hair on limbs, lack of muscle tone, thin and often dry skin, sunken eyes, dry and lacklustre hair, distended stomach and unexplained general fatigue;

- In young women, the presence of secondary amenorrhoea (the cessation of menstruation after it has been established).

Physical investigations include blood tests, electrocardiography, radiological assessment and ultrasound scans. Diagnosis and treatment can sometimes be complicated by existing chronic illnesses, such as diabetes, as the individual could be tempted to restrict insulin intake in order to lose calories. Also, the symptoms of organic intestinal disorder may occasionally hide the psychological condition.

The physical and psychological implications

Emotional distress is common in anorexia sufferers and can range from anxiety and low mood symptoms to chronic depression. The longer the young person suffers with the condition, the more likely emotional and social difficulties are to increase. These can range from an inability to care for oneself adequately, reducing or completely stopping leisure activities, giving up on educational goals and dreams, and loss of personal autonomy. These can have a profound effect on the young person's quality of life, increasing their level of dependency and the importance they place on the eating disorder. There is some evidence to suggest that depression and other mental health conditions such as OCD are more common in anorexia nervosa sufferers. Depression, for example, is a common comorbid diagnosis, with rates of up to 63 per cent in some studies (Herzog et al., 1992 cited in NICE Guidance, 2004), while OCD has been found to be present in 35 per cent of patients with anorexia nervosa (Rastam, 1992 cited in NICE Guidance, 2004).

The physical damage that anorexia nervosa inflicts upon a sufferer is significant, both in the short and long term, occurring as a consequence both of the effects of starvation and of purging behaviours. It can include:

- Damage to the musculoskeletal system, with loss of muscle strength (even the heart muscle is affected), loss of bone density and an increased risk of osteoporosis in later life, particularly in young women.

- The stress placed on the endocrine system impacts on key organs, causing a raised risk of infertility, polycystic ovaries and loss of bone mineralization.

- Where anorexia has disrupted puberty in both boys and girls, development of secondary sexual characteristics can be impaired and growth can be stunted permanently.

- Disorders in the reproductive hormones (low LH and FSH), suppressed TSH, growth hormone resistance and raised cortisol levels.

- The effects of purging and habitual vomiting (more common and profound in sufferers of bulimia nervosa) can include tooth enamel erosion, which in severe cases leads to the sufferer losing a whole set of teeth, or painful and unsightly teeth that can effect a young person's self-esteem and social confidence.

- The volume of the brain is reduced – the brain literally shrinks, and structural damage can be caused in adolescence. Cognitive development and brain function may be affected by both short- and long-term extreme weight loss in children.

- There is some suggestion that social skills are impaired and can lead to communication issues and an inability to engage in intimate relationships.

- The disruptions to day-to-day living and the disturbance caused by lengthy hospitalizations can damage education and employment prospects.

> (Goldbloom & Kennedy, 1995 cited in
> NICE Guidance, 2004)

Treatments and responses

Anorexia nervosa is treated primarily as a mental health problem, although the physical symptoms of the condition obviously need to be addressed simultaneously. Treatments focus on getting the young person to eat healthily, bolstered by dietary supplements, whilst also addressing the underlying psychological issues relating to self-perception (particularly body image) and raising self-esteem. If a young person is seriously ill and the signs of anorexia nervosa are acute, they can be sectioned under the Mental Health Act (1983) and admitted to hospital for compulsory treatment. In extreme cases, force feeding to prevent death is a possibility under the Mental Health Act (1983) and the Children's Act (1989).

Psychological treatments can be delivered on a 1:1 basis, in small groups or with family members present. This type of treatment aims to reduce the risk of harm from the illness, encourage weight gain and healthy eating, and reduce other symptoms related to the eating disorder. It can include:

- Cognitive analytic therapy (CAT)

- Cognitive behaviour therapy (CBT)

- Interpersonal therapy (IPT)

- Focal psychodynamic therapy

- Family therapy

Medication may also be part of the treatment plan and could involve anti-depressants. As anorexia sufferers are more likely to suffer from heart conditions the young person may need to have an electrocardiograph (ECG).

Prognosis for young people presenting with anorexia nervosa

It is difficult to make generalizations regarding the prognosis for young people suffering from anorexia nervosa. Those who have had a rapid and early onset experience of the condition can make a full recovery from the initial episode. The prognosis is also better where early physical and psychosocial development has previously been healthy, and where there is an identified precipitating nega-tive life event, such as the death of a close relative or parental divorce (North et al., 1997 cited in NICE, 2004). In these cases and where onset of the eating disorder is prepubertal, physical implications such as stunted growth and puber-tal delay are usually fully reversible. For others, where the onset of the eating disorder is more difficult to attribute to any specific event or trauma, but where the young person may have presented with earlier social difficulties or abnormal personality development, the prognosis is often less positive and the individual may go on to suffer from the condition well into middle age (Gowers et al., 1991 cited in NICE, 2004).

Bulimia nervosa

Bulimia nervosa is an eating disorder which prevents the individual from being able to maintain a 'normal' eating pattern. An individual with the condition becomes increasingly unable to relate normally to food and develops a depend-ency on a cycle of bingeing and purging. Typically, they alternate between the desperate activity of binge eating and a subsequent state of panic, accompanied by the need to purge themselves of what they have just eaten. Sufferers either make themselves vomit and/or use laxatives and/or diuretics to rid themselves of the food they have consumed. Some people do not purge themselves but have a period of excessive fasting or exercise to compensate for their overeat-ing. Bulimia nervosa is five times more common in young people aged 10 to 25 than anorexia nervosa, but is extremely rare in younger children. Most young people presenting with bulimia nervosa are at the upper end of the age group and may be deemed young adults rather than adolescents (AYPH, 2013).

A pre-existing anorexic illness may be part of the young person's history. Where this is not the case the development of the disorder is essentially similar to that of anorexia nervosa, often arising from a background of dietary controls or attempts to restrict food consumption. In bulimia nervosa, however, dietary control cannot be maintained and is disrupted by episodes of reactive binge eating. As a consequence, a bulimic young person will, therefore, maintain a weight, usually within the normal range, which can make it more difficult for family members or teachers to identify. The young person becomes a victim of a vicious cycle of attempted dieting, binge eating and purging, often on a daily basis. Food, and thinking about food, dominates the sufferer's life. Sufferers can be secretive about their condition and make attempts to hide the evidence or prefer to eat in private, avoiding social situations that involve food (NICE, 2004).

Young people with bulimia nervosa do not tend to disclose their behaviour willingly or seek out treatment. The condition appears to be culturally 'less valued' than anorexia nervosa, by both the medical profession and the media. Indeed, binge eating and purging are commonly associated with extreme feelings of guilt and shame in the sufferer. Media representations of the condition involve sensationalizing the 'guilty secret battles' of celebrities with bulimia, where the individual has 'admitted' or 'confessed'. A young person's reluctance to seek treatment may also arise from the fear that they will be stopped from vomiting and purging and then left to face the consequences of their binge eating – excessive weight gain. They prefer the 'feeling of control' that the purging or excessive fasting gives them than the 'unknown' presented by confronting the issue (NICE, 2004).

Other signs to be aware of in bulimia nervosa

- Mood disturbance is extremely common

- Symptoms of anxiety and tension are frequently experienced

- Self-denigrating thoughts may develop out of disgust at overeating or purging

- Low self-esteem and physical self-loathing may in some be rooted in the past experience of physical or sexual abuse

- Self-harm, commonly by scratching or cutting, is common

- A significant proportion of those with bulimia nervosa have a history of disturbed interpersonal relationships with poor impulse control

- Some sufferers will also abuse alcohol and other drugs.

(NICE, 2004).

Treatments and responses

Young people suffering with bulimia nervosa could be offered cognitive behaviour therapy (CBT) adapted to their age and the specifics of the problem. This could include the whole family if deemed appropriate. Older adolescents could be offered medication as an alternative, or in addition to CBT, and a self-help programme. Anti-depressants known as selective serotonin reuptake inhibitors (SSRIs) – and in particular fluoxetine (Prozac) – are most often chosen for treating bulimia nervosa. Studies on adult sufferers of bulimia nervosa have demonstrated some success in reducing the number of times the sufferer is binge eating and purging; however, there is no evidence to date that anti-depressants are effective in adolescents (McCann, 1990; Mitchell, 1990; Pope, 1983 and Walsh 1991; all cited in Nice guidance, 2004 pp. 128–130).

Other health implications of bulimia nervosa

For a small but significant number of people, bulimia nervosa can lead to serious physical problems, such as dehydration and changes in the chemical balance in their body that can result in heart and other physical problems. If vomiting is frequent, or the individual is taking large quantities of laxatives, a blood test may be taken to check fluid levels and chemical balance. Most treatment is undertaken as an outpatient. Any psychological treatment given for bulimia usually lasts for at least 6 months. People with additional problems, such as serious drug or alcohol misuse, are less likely to improve by just following a standard treatment, and it is often necessary to adapt the treatment to meet the needs of the patient. Very few people with bulimia nervosa need hospital treatment, and are usually only admitted if they are at risk of harming themselves physically. If they are admitted it should be into a specialist unit experienced in treating people with bulimia nervosa.

Obesity – when is an eating disorder not an eating disorder?

Anorexia nervosa and bulimia nervosa are both classified as 'eating disorders'. Obesity, in contrast, is rarely, if ever, described as such. This is despite the fact that it can be equally serious in its health implications. Obesity is, nonetheless, regarded by most authorities as a major public health issue, not just in the UK, but globally.

The main measurement scale used to assess body weight is the 'Body Mass Index' (BMI), a scale in which body mass is assessed in relation to height. The basic equation involves dividing the person's weight by the square of their height in metres (kg/m^2). The World Health Organization's definition of being 'overweight' is a BMI of 25 or more, and the definition of 'obesity' is a BMI of 30 or more. A raised BMI is a major risk factor for the development of a variety of diseases, including cardiovascular disease, type 2 diabetes and many cancers, raising the risk of premature mortality and long-term health problems. The impact of being overweight or obese on the emotional health and well-being of young people growing up in the increasingly 'body image' obsessed popular culture of twenty-first-century life can also be devastating. Being overweight or obese in adolescence is associated with a significant reduction in the quality of life and places the individual at a greater risk of teasing, bullying and social isolation (WHO, 2012).

Obesity in the UK, as in other affluent countries, has been caused primarily by behavioural and environmental change across society (NHF, 2007). Historically, the rich were fat and the poor were thin, but in recent decades this trend has been reversed. The problem appears to be most acute in those countries with greater levels of inequality – including the UK. Childhood obesity prevalence in the UK is highest in the most deprived areas. The National Child Measurement Programme (NCMP, 2011–2012) found, for example, that child obesity prevalence in the most deprived 10 per cent of the population is approximately twice that among the least deprived 10 per cent. These findings suggest that the inequalities gap in child obesity in the UK is continuing to widen.

Some of this pattern appears related to the impact of economic austerity. Evidence from DEFRA (2013) suggests that recent rises in food prices have resulted in a marked reduction in the consumption of fruit and vegetables. Most concerning is that it is children and young people in particular that have started to eat less fruit and vegetables. In 2011 DEFRA reported that only 18 per cent managed to eat five portions a day. The average daily consumption of 'five a day' for girls aged 11–18 years was reported to be 2.8 per cent in the UK; and for boys of the same age the intake averaged 3 per cent (DH/FSA, 2011). The figures also showed that 6.6 per cent of adults and 4.7 per cent of children have no fruit or vegetables at all in their diet (DEFRA, 2013).

Rising food prices and falling incomes are not the whole story however. Research over recent decades has confirmed what many people already intuitively knew; that across the population – men and women, young and old, rich and poor have been getting fatter. The global prevalence of obesity has increased at such a rate in the past 30 years that the WHO (2012) estimates that the number of overweight children aged under 18 years is now over 170 million worldwide.

A significant factor underlying this is the rise of what has been described as the 'obesogenic environment'. Obesity levels are rising in the Western world because, in the average lifestyle, food is plentiful whilst there is less need for physical activity in our day-to-day lives. We live in paradoxical times; where parts of the world are literally starving to death, whilst other parts are literally gorging themselves to early deaths on high calorie, high fat and highly salted foods. The only thing these two worlds share is that they are both suffering from malnutrition: one with too little to eat, whilst the other, too much of the wrong kind of cheap, over-processed, energy-dense, nutritionally poor food (Pearce et al., 2008).

Body weight is determined primarily by the simple equation that the daily calories consumed must not exceed the calories expended by the needs of the body in simply living and undertaking daily activity. Nutrition experts and dietitians would emphasize that it is also the nutritional quality of what we are consuming as well as the quantity of what we eat that is having a profound effect on our weight, quality of life and well-being.

The prevalence and impact of obesity

Data from the Health Survey for England (HSE) demonstrates that the prevalence of childhood obesity increased between 1995 and 2004, with a levelling off in the last decade for 11- to 15-year-olds. However, the prevalence of obesity is still increasing year-on-year among boys and girls in Year 6, 10- to 11-year-olds – the pre-teenage group. In 2011 a third of 11-year-old children in England were categorized as overweight or obese. NCMP data showed that 33.4 per cent of Year 6 children are overweight or obese, equalling the percentage rate for children in 2010. The programme demonstrates that, since 2006, obesity levels have risen in primary school leavers, with a figure of 19 per cent in 2011, compared to 17.5 per cent in 2007. Overall, the percentage of overweight children has remained roughly level at an average of 14.4 per cent over the past 5 years. Levels of obesity also appear to be higher in urban areas compared to rural areas for both YR and Y6 children, as was the case in previous years of the NCMP. The obesity prevalence is also significantly higher than the national average for children in both school years in the ethnic groups 'Asian or Asian British', 'Any Other Ethnic Group' and 'Black or Black British' and for the ethnic group 'Mixed' in Year 6.

Obesity significantly increases the risk of developing a range of serious health problems, including hypertension, late onset diabetes, cardiovascular disease, gallbladder disease and some cancers, in later life. Current trends in childhood obesity are predicted to lead to a shorter life expectancy for today's children compared with their parents – the first reversal in life expectancy since the nineteenth century. This projection is one that grabs the attention of the media and public health policy makers alike, and is the key driver behind the strategies and interventions being put in place in an attempt to reverse this trend. There are also major social and economic implications, however. The possible future costs of managing a widespread epidemic of obesity-related ill health, such as diabetes and cardiovascular disease, for example, are enormous, and some suggest potentially bankrupting for the NHS. Type 2 diabetes, the form strongly associated with obesity, is also a major cause of blindness and amputations in later life, with significant implications across society, ranging from people's capacity to work, travel and require support systems and resources (Akabas, Lederman and Moore, 2012).

Responses and strategies

Obesity is regarded as the most serious threat to the physical health and well-being of children and young people in the UK. Millions have been spent on health promotion campaigns to improve the diets and increase physical activity rates of children and young people in the UK. There is very little evidence, however, to suggest these have been effective as yet. As the discourse surrounding the concept of an 'obesogenic environment' gathers pace many are calling for wider political and economic solutions. Ebbling et al. (2002), for example, have called for a 'common sense approach' involving fundamental changes to the social environment, including a tax on fast food and soft drinks. Tackling the powerful global food corporations and their marketing techniques with clear legislative directives is the course of action that many campaigners are calling for, but governments currently appear reluctant to follow. This has not always been the case, however, and before we consider recent government strategies and policies, it is informative to take a brief look at this history.

Historically, the most significant intervention by government in the eating habits of the nation was the war-time rationing and supplementation of children's diet with vitamin C and cod liver oil during the Second World War. Whilst in part a measure to ensure there was enough food to go around, rationing also aimed at ensuring that the population was as fit and healthy as possible, and able to take its role in Britain's war machine. School meals became available to all school children, 14 per cent of which were available free of charge. The rest were charged at the cost price of the ingredients. Local authorities received subsidies to cover a substantial proportion of the cost of school meals (Gillard, 2003). The 1944 Education Act made the provision of school meals a statutory duty for local authorities.

An increasing body of knowledge and understanding around the nutritional needs of children supported the government's direction of increasing involvement in improving their diets. The 1945 Labour government brought in universal free school milk in an effort to improve the calcium intake of the young. Food rationing lasted until 1954, and some make the claim that young people's diets in the 1950s were actually healthier as a result of rationing than their modern day counterparts (Meikle, 1999).

Successive Labour and Conservative governments in the 1960s and 1970s shared a consensus of opinion that the provision of a nutritionally balanced school meal was too socially valuable to interfere with, but neither did much more to improve the diets of the young. Indeed both continuously took steps to reduce government spending on public services. Most controversial of all was the ending of universal free school milk by Margaret Thatcher as Minister for Education, a step which earned her the title 'Margaret Thatcher, Milk Snatcher'.

In 1979, Margaret Thatcher became Prime Minister, and the reduction of public spending began in earnest in 1980 with the abolition of statutory nutritional standards for school meals and the obligation of local authorities to provide a school meal service. The Thatcher governments also introduced the policy of commercial competitive tendering, which compelled local authorities to select the 'most competitive' – inevitably meaning the cheapest – catering service available to run their school meal provision. This had a serious effect on the nutritional quality of school meals, as many schools switched to a 'free choice' cafeteria style service, where cost-cutting measures and the need to make a profit meant that children ate a daily diet of burgers and chips, or what the campaigning chef Jamie Oliver later labelled, a diet of 'turkey twizzlers and chips'. The Social Security Act of 1986 also meant that thousands of children lost their right to a free school meal.

These policy changes were part of the changing social and economic structure of Britain; a transformation that led to children's nutritional health becoming further compromised. Technological changes brought an increasing dependency on freezer and TV dinner meals. Growing numbers of families needed both parents to work, and often found it increasingly difficult to find the time to plan and cook. This era also saw the relentless rise of fast food culture. Meanwhile, in schools the selling of school fields to raise money, the introduction of the National Curriculum and the abolition of Home Economics contributed to leaving many young people with fewer opportunities for physical activity and less understanding of the importance of cooking and healthy diets.

Recent strategies addressing obesity and nutrition

The so-called New Labour government, elected in 1997, attempted to address the 'new' public health issue of obesity specifically, and poor diet among young people generally. Groups such as the National Heart Forum and the National Medical Council argued that the state of children's and young people's diets amounted to a public health time bomb, and a number of charities launched campaigns promoting reduced intake of high salt and sugar foods, and the consumption of fresh fruit and vegetables. The government introduced a wave of initiatives aimed at halting the rise in childhood obesity rates; all of which were integral to the government's Every Child Matters (2003) with its five outcomes:

- Be healthy

- Be safe

- Enjoy and achieve

- Make a positive contribution

- Economic well-being.

In 1997, the Food Standards Agency (FSA), in partnership with the Department of Health (DOH), undertook a survey of young people's diet and nutrition which confirmed that they were eating less fruit and vegetables, consuming more junk food and participating in less physical activity than ever before. This report confirmed also that it was children from deprived backgrounds who had the worst diets, consumed the most sugar, fat and salt and exercised the least. Whilst the government responded to the survey by asking the food industry to 'tone down' their advertising of junk food and urged them to promote healthy lifestyles instead, the industry's response was decidedly cool. It has been argued since that one of the most significant failings of the New Labour government in terms of childhood health was its reluctance to regulate the food industry.

The key initiatives that shaped government responses to childhood obesity between 1997 and 2010 included:

The National School Fruit Scheme – The New Labour government's NHS Plan made a commitment to develop a National five-a-day Programme to increase fruit and vegetable consumption. The National School Fruit Scheme (NSFS), launched in 2004, entitled all infants to a free piece of fruit each school day. Evidence from evaluations of the national scheme supported campaigners' requests that the scheme should be extended to cover the 7-11-year-old age group. The current freeze on public spending makes this very unlikely, however, although individual schools do opt to use their central funding to roll out the programme to older pupils. Britain is one of only four EU member states that have opted out of the European Commission's funding scheme for free fruit and vegetables to all primary school-aged children, prompting dismay among healthy eating campaigners.

Public Service Agreements (PSA) –Targets for physical activity – In 2007, the New Labour government's Comprehensive Spending Review set out new national indicators that would measure the progress of targets around childhood obesity at a local level. Targets for improving physical activity rates of children and young people were among the mandatory indicators for measuring the progress of local authorities. These targets gave the School Sports Partnership Programme some authority when it came to working with schools to improve the quality and accessibility of their PE lessons and physical activity opportunities (PE and sport strategy for young people, DCSF, 2008).

Extended Schools – In 'Extended schools: building on experience' (Department for Children, Schools and Families, 2007), the government set out a programme of extended services by schools for children, young people and their families to be met by 2010. This could include: childcare services, a wide range of after-school activities, particularly sport, parenting support and community access to facilities.

Children and play – As we have seen in other chapters, there has been rising concern in recent years about children's reduced opportunities to play and the impact this is having on childhood obesity rates. 'The play strategy' aimed to create safe, welcoming, interesting, accessible and free places to play in every residential community. Children and young people had a role in its planning. It was backed by £235 million of dedicated investment (Department for Children, Schools and Families, 2008d). A flurry of other strategies was introduced at this time in an attempt to address the issues around children and play, which included:

- Time for play (Department for Culture, Media and Sport, 2006)

- Getting serious about play (Department for Culture, Media and Sport, 2004)

- Playing to win: a new era for sport (Department for Culture, Media and Sport, 2008)

- Before, during and after: making the most of the London 2012 games (Department for Culture, Media and Sport, 2008)

- Sport England strategy 2008–2011 (Sport England, 2008)

- Free swimming for the under 16s, a cross-government initiative announced in July 2008.

The School Travel Plan – National policies on active travel aimed to reduce car use and promote sustainable modes of travel. The New Labour government demanded that each local education authority should have a sustainable mode of travel strategy to meet the school travel needs of their area (HM Government, 2006). A joint Department for Children, Schools and Families (DoCSF) and Department for Transport (DoT) target was set for all schools to have an approved school travel plan that addressed sustainability and pupil health and fitness by March 2010 (Department for Education and Skills, 2006). This was supported by the 'Travelling to school initiative' (Department for Transport, 2005) and the 'Sustainable schools for pupils, communities and the environment' (Department for Education and Skills, 2006). Wider initiatives supported the school-based travel plan, such as the DoT's 'home zone' initiative, which aimed to make streets more attractive to pedestrians and cyclists by introducing ways to reduce traffic speed (traffic calming measures), parking areas, benches and play areas (Department for Transport, 2005). The National Healthy Schools Programme, before its demise in 2011, required all schools to have an up-to-date travel plan to achieve healthy schools status.

National Child Measurement Programme (NCMP) – The National Child Measurement Programme was launched in 2005 to gather data on children in Year R and Year 6 of primary school. Robust data is seen as key to supporting the efforts to tackle childhood obesity. It is this data that will continue to inform both national and local responses to the issue of childhood obesity. The frustration for health professionals working with children and young people around obesity, both when the programme was initiated and today, is the fact that more time and investment is spent on collecting the data than on actual interventions to respond effectively to what the data is telling us. To date there is little evidence that the NCMP is having a positive impact on childhood obesity rates, other than by helping to raise the profile of childhood obesity as a key issue. An evaluation of the NCMP (Coram, 2011) focused on the delivery of the programme rather than its impact on childhood obesity rates.

Change4Life Programme – The Change4Life Programme was the government's own public health programme. It used social marketing approaches to campaign on the causes of obesity. Although aimed at the whole population, it had children and families as a key target group. It used an integrated marketing approach to encourage families to make small, manageable changes to their eating and exercise habits that together could make a difference to their weight and fitness levels. It focused on six key behaviours:

- Five-a-day – encouraging families to increase their daily consumption of fruit and vegetables
- Watch the salt – a campaign to reduce salt intake
- Cut back on the fat – information on how to reduce fat content of meals
- Sugar swaps – healthier alternatives to sugar
- Reducing alcohol consumption
- Get going every day – how to incorporate activity into your day easily and cheaply

National Healthy Schools Programme – The National Healthy Schools Programme was launched in 1999, heralding a new partnership between health and education at both a national and local level. 'Healthy Schools' was an integral part of the Children's Plan (DCSF, 2007) and the Department of Health's *Healthy Weight, Healthy Lives* (DOH, 2008). Addressing childhood obesity by promoting healthy eating and physical activity were central for schools looking to achieve the status of a National Healthy Schools Award. Schools were also encouraged (although not required) to have healthy lunch box policies, and to work closely with children, young people and their families to promote healthy lunch boxes alongside promoting the uptake of the new nutritionally balanced school meals.

The Coalition government elected in 2010 cut all national funding for the Healthy Schools programme in 2011, and whilst the toolkit to support schools in promoting health and well-being is still available, many fear the momentum has now been lost under the increased demands on schools to meet exam targets above all else.

Non-government initiatives to tackle obesity

Alongside the government initiatives the voluntary sector has also focused on the health and well-being of children and young people. Initiatives in recent years include:

- **Play England** – part of the National Children's Bureau; it provides advice and support to promote good practice. It also works to ensure that policy makers, planners and the public recognize the importance of play.

- **Youth Sport Trust** – supports the nationwide network of school sports partnerships. It also works with underrepresented groups through programmes such as Girls in Sport, Living for Sport, YoUR Activity, TOP Activity and the Playground to Podium framework for young disabled people.

- **The British Heart Foundation** – runs initiatives and provides physical activity resources.

- **The Fitness Industry Association** – runs 'go' (an outreach programme) and the 'Adopt a School' programme. Both were developed to help build stronger links between the fitness industry and schools. 'Go' also aims to help teenage girls (aged 15 and 16) to understand the benefits of being active and show that it can be fun. 'Adopt a school' targets children aged 10 and 11 in the final year of primary school.

The examples given here are by no means exhaustive, and demonstrate the range of policies, initiatives and resources undertaken by various voluntary organizations to try to increase activity rates in children and young people.

Critical observers have been quick to point out, however, that despite the good intentions, and whilst many of them do focus on sport and sporting opportunities, only a minority appear to promote lifetime physical activity or focus on lifestyle and unstructured activities (Cale and Harris, 2006). Recent research into regular, routine exercise such as walking and the commute to school or work suggests that efforts to promote changes in lifestyle habits could have a more profound impact on obesity levels than the campaigns to get people engaging in organized weekly exercise classes.

The 'austerity agenda' and its impact on government's response to young people's obesity

In 2004, the New Labour government made a pledge to halt childhood obesity by 2010, but as the extent and depth of the problem became clear this was later shifted to 2020. The Foresight Report (2007) warned that, such was the severity of the issue, it would take at least 30 years and over £45 billion a year to turn it around. Campaigners feared that shifting the target would result in focus on the issue drifting and losing momentum, and to many it sounded like an admission of defeat. With hindsight it could also be seen as initiating the change of policy direction of the incoming Coalition government in 2010.

The Coalition government initiated a programme of severe cuts in public spending that has fundamentally changed the way childhood obesity is now addressed. The incoming Health Minister, Andrew Lansley, spoke of a 'new approach to public health', with the government asking charities, local authorities and the commercial sector to take a much greater role. This reflected the adoption of the so-called nudge theory, as distinct from a direct government-led response to obesity. Critics argued that it effectively meant giving up on challenging the 'obesogenic environment' and government regulation of the food industry, placing responsibility instead back onto individuals and families.

The Coalition government's key policies included:

- *Public Health White Paper: Healthy Lives, Healthy People (Nov 2010)* – This announced that, from April 2013, tackling obesity would become the responsibility of local authorities.

- *A Call to Action on Obesity (October 2011)* – This set out two national ambitions. First, a downward trend in the level of excess weight averaged across all adults by 2020; and second, a sustained downward trend in the level of excess weight in children by 2020. 'A Call for Action' confirmed the Coalition government's acceptance of the analysis of the Foresight Report, 2007, commissioned by the previous government, focusing on a 'life-course approach' – from pre-conception through pregnancy, infancy, early years, childhood, adolescence, to adulthood and preparing for older age. The government is also continuing to support the NCMP so that local areas have information to plan and commission local services and support local authorities to build on this evidence base through the work of the National Obesity Observatory. It goes on to state its intention to work with the food and drink industry, as part of what it calls the 'Public Health Responsibility Deal'.

- *The New School Food Plan (July 2013)* – An initiative by chefs, Henry Dimbleby and John Vincent, essentially revamping previous campaigns to improve school meals, and reminiscent of Jamie Oliver's 'Million' Campaign. The School Food Trust is also aiming to bring back cooking to the school curriculum and improve the quality of school meals.

- *Free school meals for infant school-aged children (Sept 2014)* – A Liberal Democrat-led initiative to provide free school meals for all children aged 4–7 years. Welcomed by many school meal campaigners, but only cautiously welcomed by schools due to the difficulties of implementing it – including staffing issues, lack of space and lack of time to get the sheer volume of pupils through in a lunchtime.

Some conclusions about obesity and nutrition

The fundamental difference between the New Labour approach to obesity and that of the subsequent Coalition and Conservative governments was in how these strategies are funded and resourced. The 'new approach' to public health is largely dependent on the voluntary sector filling the gap left by the cuts to public services, together with voluntary contributions from the food industry, and the hope that by 'nudging' the general public towards healthier lifestyle habits the waistlines of the nation will correspondingly reduce.

This change of approach will be discussed further in Chapter 10, when we discuss health promotion strategies aimed at young people. Any meaningful government response to the issue of obesity will need, however, to be multifaceted to deal with the complexities of the issue. There is no simple solution. As Sir David King, the chief scientific adviser to the government, commented in 2007, 'the nation had "sleepwalked" into it [obesity] because our hunter-gatherer biology was out of step with the technological convenience age; we were programmed to eat as if we did not know where the next meal was coming from. If we just behave normally we will become obese' (BBC News Channel, 17 October 2007).

Although individuals do make their own choices about their eating and exercise habits, it is, we would argue, hopelessly naive and unfair to lay responsibility entirely with individuals and families to address the obesity crisis, when it is clear that so many of the economic, social and cultural changes of the last 50 years have had a profound impact on our relationship with food and physical activity. Changes in many different areas of society are necessary, from the planning and design of towns and transport systems, to encouraging healthier food production and consumption. Only then perhaps will we be able to have a real chance of halting the rise of childhood obesity, and of ensuring that young people have optimum opportunities for good nutrition.

Suggested Further Reading

All Party Parliamentary Group on Body Image. (2012) *Reflections on Body Image*. London: All Party Parliamentary Group on Body Image/YMCA.

HMSO (2007) *Foresight Report: Tackling Obesities: Future Choices. Project Report*. (2nd edition) Crown Copyright.

King, N. A., Hills, A. P., and Byrne, N. M. (2007) *Children, Obesity and Exercise: Studies in the Prevention, Treatment and Management of Childhood and Adolescent Obesity*. London: Routledge.

Mazzocchi, M. (2009) *Fat Economics: Nutrition, Health, and Economic Policy*. Oxford: Oxford University Press.

NICE (2005) *Obsessive compulsive disorder and body dysmorphic disorder*: treatment. NICE Guidelines [CG31] November 2005.

Shipton, G. (2004) *Working with Eating Disorders*. Basingstoke: Palgrave Macmillan.

Vash, P. D. (ed.) (2015) *The Childhood Obesity Epidemic; Why Are Our Children Obese and What Can We Do about It?* Apple Academic Press.

Wykes, M. and Gunter, B. (2004) *The Media and Body Image: If Looks Could Kill*. Sage.

9

SUBSTANCE USE AND MISUSE

In this chapter we will look at young people's use of substances and some of the responses. The term 'substances' will be used here as a general term to include substances that are legal in the UK, such as alcohol and tobacco, and those that are illegal, such as cannabis and cocaine. The Home Office drugs strategy (Home Office, 2010, p. 8) states that the rate of drug use by young people in the UK has fallen by a third in the past decade. This suggests an encouraging picture. But when placed within a European context, the reality looks somewhat less positive. Rates of so-called binge drinking and cannabis use by young people in the UK, for example, are among the highest in Europe.

When parents approach schools and youth organizations for support and advice their anxiety tends to be focused on what they see as 'hard' drugs like cocaine, heroin and ecstasy. The evidence suggests that more attention actually needs to be given to the health impacts of alcohol and tobacco. This highlights an important distinction between substance use which is seen as socially acceptable (if not necessarily desirable) and substance use, or 'misuse', that is, for one reason or another, deemed unacceptable. Substance misuse is officially defined as:

> ...intoxication by – or regular excessive consumption of and/or dependence on – psychoactive substances, leading to social, psychological, physical or legal problems. It includes problematic use of both legal and illegal drugs (including alcohol when used in combination with other substances). (National Institute of Care Excellence [NICE] 2007a, 1a, p. 5)

The key health-related issues are seen as harmfulness and dependence, and it is claimed that this is what underlies the distinction in law between legal and illegal substances, a distinction based on two key factors:

1   Drugs and substances are deemed illicit because they cause addiction and associated health issues of a severity which means they are a serious societal concern;

2   Illegal drugs cause crime and are particularly associated with social unrest
    and violent crime.

                                                                (Boland, 2008)

Given what we know about the relative harm caused to individuals and society by
alcohol as compared, for instance, with cannabis, these are arguable points, and
we will return to question them further below, but initially, a key question to ask is:
'Why do young people use or misuse substances?'

     We will explore some of the theories about motivations for substance use/
misuse, and their implications for treatment and responses later. But for now we
can say that the answers are likely to be a mixture of the following:

● pleasure and enjoyment;

● self-medication and/or escapism;

● peer pressure and/or social acceptance;

● the 'frisson' and 'glamour' of danger and rebellion;

● a shortcut to 'adult' self-image and identity.

These factors are important to understand if we are to design health promotion
strategies aimed at reducing harm and minimizing risk. We also need to understand why some young people are more susceptible to using, and misusing,
substances, whether legal or illegal. The risks can, of course, be considerable.
They include:

● poisoning from overdose and/or taking poorly manufactured illegal drugs or
  toxic substances, whether legal or illegal. Around 13,000 alcohol-related
  hospital admissions are reported each year for young people in the UK
  (Home Office, 2010);

● gaining a criminal record and bad reputation which can be difficult to shake
  off – potentially leading to social and educational exclusion, unemployment,
  social marginalization, loss of family support, and even homelessness, if use
  and dependence is intense and prolonged;

● cumulative damage to physical and mental health over the long term, particularly with substances that lead to addiction and dependence;

● exposure to other risks, including early or unwanted sex – and the accompa-
  nying risks of sexually transmitted infection, unwanted pregnancy and exposure to violence and/or crime.

Addiction and dependence are complex phenomena, involving a mix of physiological, neurological, psychological and sociocultural factors. But the defining

aspect is that an addicted person begins to lose control over their use of the substance and develops a compulsive need to keep taking it in order to function and cope with life. The NHS defines addiction as:

> ...not having control over doing taking or using something to the point that it may be harmful. (National Treatment Agency for Substance Misuse, 2010)

Addiction leads to dependence, which is defined as:

> ...the compulsion to continue taking a drug in order to feel good and to avoid feeling bad. (National Treatment Agency for Substance Misuse, 2010)

We will look at addiction and dependence issues in more detail below. First, let us look briefly at the historical and cultural background to substance use in the UK.

A historical and cultural perspective

There is a tendency to view substance use as a particular problem of the modern world. In fact, taking mind-altering substances is as old as humankind. The origins of human consumption of substances certainly go back to prehistoric hunter-gatherer societies, for pleasure, medicine, and religious and spiritual ceremonies and rituals. Many currently existing hunter-gatherer societies have a rich knowledge and lore surrounding mind- and performance-enhancing substances, and use them for a variety of recreational, religious and medicinal reasons (Burns, 2007).

There is a long history too of substance use, for similar reasons, in so-called civilized societies. Wine, for example, was being produced and consumed at least as early as the ancient Egyptians around 4000 BC, and its use is still included in Christian religious ceremonies – a fact that has no doubt played a large part in the acceptance and legality of alcohol in societies influenced by Christianity. Medicinal use of cannabis has been dated back to around 2737 BC in China, and its use is still regarded as having religious significance in Rastafarianism. A variety of stimulants and hallucinogenic substances have traditionally been used across Africa, Asia and South America since prehistory, including the stimulant 'ghat', unrefined versions of cocaine (in the form of coca leaves) and heroin (in the form of opium). Mushrooms inducing hallucinations and trance-like states have been widely used for centuries for religious and shamanic purposes in Northern and Western Europe (Burns, 2007; Emmet & Nice, 2006).

In European history wealthy explorers, merchants and travellers in the imperial age began recreational use of tobacco, opium, cannabis and other substances, and the 'romance' of substance use emerged. Townsend (2008) provides an interesting and concise summary of the influence of substance use on Western literature. The romantic poet Samuel Coleridge, for example, wrote one of his most famous pieces, 'Kubla Khan', after taking laudanum in 1797 – a substance that eventually killed him in 1834. Robert Louis Stevenson wrote the iconic *The Strange Case of Dr Jekyll and Mr Hyde* (1866) during a six-day cocaine binge. And, of course, there are the famously hallucinogenic tales of *Alice in Wonderland* and *Alice Through the Looking Glass* by Lewis Carroll.

The chemical extraction of active substances from their 'raw' versions began in the West in the nineteenth century, leading to the development of drugs, such as morphine and lignocaine, for medicinal use. The production and distribution of these and other powerful substances was largely unregulated until after the Second World War, however, and they often appeared in popular over-the-counter medicines, such as cough linctus, into the 1940s and 1950s.

During the 1960s, patterns of substance use became more strongly associated with youth culture, becoming linked to a romantic spirit of rebellion and challenge to authority. Music, art and fashion were heavily influenced during the so-called psychedelic era in the late 1960s. The romantic image was quickly shattered, however, by high-profile causalities such as Janis Joplin, Jimi Hendrix and Jim Morrison, and the notorious 'Manson murders' in California. There was also increasing concern over the uncontrolled manufacture, smuggling and selling of hard drugs, and growing links to organized crime. By the 1970s, youth culture and illegal drug use had become inextricably linked in the popular view of society (Townsend, 2008).

In the 1980s and 1990s substance use patterns changed again. A gulf opened up, for example, between rich and poor, exemplified by the use of refined cocaine as a so-called designer-drug by affluent young professionals, whilst a crudely made, highly addictive and toxic form of cocaine called 'crack' became a destructive and widespread blight in many poor communities. The 1990s also saw the rise of 'party' drugs, such as ecstasy, as part of the so-called rave culture of the time. This was paralleled by specifically teen-orientated marketing campaigns from major drinks companies of products such as 'alcopops', which blurred the distinction between soft and alcoholic drinks.

Substance use among young people today

Currently, the most commonly used substances taken by young people are alcohol, tobacco and cannabis, and current statistics show that there appears to have been a recent decline in their use. Despite this, rates of substance use by young people in the UK are amongst the highest in Europe (ESPAD Report, 2011).

We will now look in more detail at the nature and health impact of a variety of substances, beginning with alcohol.

Alcohol

Alcohol is a legal substance that has a range of short- and long-term side effects. It is essentially a toxin and an addictive depressant that can reduce inhibitions in the short term and make the drinker feel more sociable. It is heavily marketed to young people by drinks companies using advertising campaigns which emphasize the enhancement of social and sexual desirability, and its centrality to the 'party' experience. Some forms of alcoholic drinks are designed specifically to blur the distinction between 'soft' and alcoholic drinks – as with so-called alcopops. Other forms are marketed as the marks of a sophisticated and affluent adult identity (Leyshon, 2011).

Alcohol use can be particularly dangerous to young people's health and well-being. Over the longer term, regular consumption of alcohol can disrupt sleep patterns, increase the risk of various cancers, heart attack, liver problems, reduce fertility and lead to high blood pressure. Historically, admissions to hospital for liver diseases linked to alcohol consumption were predominantly in the 50+ age group, but there has recently been an increase in the number of people dying of liver disease in their 20s and 30s. NHS figures show that the number of young drinkers with serious liver problems has risen by more than 50 per cent in the last decade (NHS Information Centre, 2011).

Binge drinking – that is, drinking excessively during a relatively short period of time, and perhaps repeatedly over a weekend or the duration of a holiday – is particularly associated with young people in the UK. It is also linked with risky sexual behaviour and increased risks of becoming involved in accidents and crime (Lynch and Blake, 2004; ACMD, 2006).

Drinking alcohol is also linked to the use of other substances and to problem behaviour patterns both at school and at home. Young people who drink alcohol are more likely to smoke regularly, take other substances and to have truanted from school. There are clear links also to poverty and being in care (NHS, 2010). There are some encouraging signs among younger adolescents, however. Recent research suggests a steady decline in the number of school-aged pupils between the ages of 11 and 15 who drink alcohol. A marked decline was reported, for example, in an NHS study that found that 45 per cent of 11- to 15-year-olds participating stated that they had drunk alcohol at least once in their lives, compared to 61 per cent in 2003 (NCSR and NFER, 2010).

Alcohol use is more difficult to respond to than most other substances because of the distinct position it holds in UK culture, where it is widely viewed as a mainstream pleasure. Sigman (2011) argues that alcohol is the nation's drug of choice, stating:

the problem of young drinking doesn't take place in a vacuum, but with a backdrop of alcohol-adoring adults including parents, teachers, doctors, police ... and of course, celebrities. (Sigman, 2011, p. ix)

He goes on to call for more honesty about how we view alcohol and young people, suggesting that early exposure to alcohol can have direct effects on brain size, intellectual development and ability, school performance and future fertility. He calls for a complete rethink on the way we approach alcohol, with parents needing to talk to their children honestly about alcohol with support from schools and other influential sources – including the drinks industry – to do so effectively.

Tobacco

Like alcohol, tobacco is a legal substance and is one of the commonest used by young people. Tobacco contains nicotine, which is highly addictive, alongside some 4000 other chemicals which can damage the cells and systems of the body. Smoking increases the likelihood of coughs and chest infections, is linked to the amputation of around two thousand limbs each year, and is estimated to contribute to 120,000 premature deaths in the UK every year. Approximately a third of all cancer-related deaths can be attributed to smoking tobacco. It is also a risk factor for cumulative damage, increasing the likelihood in later life of strokes, heart attacks and emphysema (FRANK, 2014).

Unlike alcohol, recent decades have seen a major change in social, cultural and political attitudes towards tobacco use. It was the recognition that 'passive smoking' – inhaling the smoke from other people's cigarettes – is as bad for people's health as actually smoking the cigarette that led to this change. Smoking has been progressively banned in public spaces – pubs, restaurants, cinemas and public transport – in the UK to the point where it has become, almost, a 'pariah' activity. This has been accompanied by a progressively more aggressive ban on advertising, and a legal requirement to display prominent health warnings and graphic images of the damage to the body caused by smoking on cigarette packets. Taxation on the purchase of tobacco has also been steadily increased, raising the price substantially. Not surprisingly, there has been a downward trend in tobacco use across all age groups in the population as a result.

Among young people, smoking rates vary with age, with 12 per cent of 15-year-olds in a recent study reporting that they smoked at least once a week, compared to less than 0.5 per cent of 11-year-olds. Teenage girls are more likely to smoke regularly than boys. However, overall, there appears to be a downward trend in smoking that mirrors that of the adult population. The same study reported that 27 per cent of 11- to 15-year-old participants in the NHS study had smoked at least once in their lives, compared with 53 per cent in a 1982 NHS study (NHS, 2011).

Cannabis

Cannabis is the most widely used illegal substance in the UK amongst both adults and young people. According to the British Crime Survey (2010) cannabis remains the illegal drug most likely to be used by young people aged 16–24, with 16.1 per cent of participants in this survey stating they had used cannabis. Young people's use of cannabis tends to increase with age, with 0.2 per cent of 11-year-olds reporting using cannabis, compared to 21.1 per cent of 15-year-olds. There appears to be an overall downward trend, however, with 8.2 per cent of pupils aged 11–15 reporting using cannabis in 2010 compared with 8.9 per cent in 2009. This follows the general decline in the prevalence of cannabis use seen since 2001 in the UK (NHS, 2010).

Cannabis is used to pleasurably alter mood, but can also cause anxiety and paranoia, and it has been linked to the onset of psychosis in some young people – particularly the high-strength form known as 'skunk'. There is some debate too over its addictiveness, but it is most often taken together with tobacco, which is addictive, and which also has its own array of detrimental health effects, as outlined above (Pycroft, 2010).

Attitudes to cannabis use seem to be undergoing something of a sea-change currently. Advocates of a 'relative harm' approach to drug policy, for example, point out that cannabis use is much less socially damaging than alcohol use, both in its immediate and long-term impacts (Nutt, 2009). This was reflected for a time in the UK by a shift towards decriminalization by the New Labour government in the 1990s. This policy was fairly quickly reversed, however, due to adverse press campaigns and public pressure, demonstrating that, in the UK at least, the popular will for change is not yet in place for this shift to occur. Nonetheless, a worldwide trend towards decriminalization, and even legalization, appears to be underway, which may yet gain the same sort of momentum that the anti-tobacco campaign developed, and it will be interesting to see how this plays out in the future.

Volatile substances

For many years, this type of substance misuse was termed 'solvent abuse' but in reality it encompasses a diverse range of substances, including solvents such as glue, 'Tippex', aerosol propellants, gases and nitrates (poppers). Many of these substances are common household goods found in the cupboards and on the shelves of family homes across the UK. They are deliberately inhaled in order to get a temporary 'high', and a sense of dizziness and euphoria. However, they can also cause vomiting, blackouts, rashes, aggressive behaviour, mood swings, impaired judgement, hallucinations, severe headaches, depression, asphyxiation, coma and even death, including to first-time users (Innovation with Substance and Southampton Healthy Schools, 2011). Between 2000 and 2008 volatile substance abuse killed more 10- to 15-year-olds than all other illegal drugs combined (talktofrank.com/drug/solvent/12/08/13). Nonetheless, this is an area of substance misuse often overlooked in schools' drugs education provision.

Thankfully, it is still rare for young people to become regular abusers of VS's. The NHS 2010 study reported that 3.8 per cent of pupils aged 11–15 years reported sniffing volatile substances such as glue, gas, aerosols or other solvents, a decrease from the 5.5 per cent of pupils self-reporting in 2009. Inhaling poppers has fallen from a high of 4.8 per cent in 2007 to 1.5 per cent in 2010. Unlike other drugs, where use tends to increase with age, the sniffing of volatile substances tends to remain constant across the age groups, disappearing almost completely at 16 years of age and over. Workers in this field suggest that this is perhaps explained by the fact that users discover other 'better' and longer lasting ways of 'getting high' and 'progress' to other drugs (Innovation with Substance and Southampton Healthy Schools, 2011).

'Class A' drugs: ecstasy, cocaine, crack, heroin, LSD, methadone and magic mushrooms

The term 'Class A drugs' refers to the classification of substances in the Dangerous Drugs Act 1971. This means they are regarded as 'most harmful' in the eyes of the law. The evidence suggests that young people rarely use Class A drugs, due probably to issues around accessibility and affordability. Between 2001 and 2009, the number of school age pupils who reported taking any Class A drugs had dropped from 4 per cent to 2.4 per cent according to the NHS Survey (2010). Class A drug use gets higher, however, as we progress up the age range. According to the British Crime Survey for 2009/2010 7.3 per cent of young adults aged 16–24 had used Class A drugs in 2010 compared to 8.1 per cent in 2009. The long-term picture indicates that Class A drug use among young people has stabilized since 1996 (Home Office, 2010).

The issue of 'relative harm' referred to above in relation to cannabis also raises its head in relation to these substances. Although no one doubts the dangers and negative health impacts of using heroin, cocaine or crack, there is debate about whether substances such as ecstasy and magic mushrooms should be put in the same category. It is unlikely that the legal status of these substances will change any time soon in the UK, however, but it is worth noting that some countries, such as Portugal, are experimenting with radical shifts in policy which are being watched with great interest.

In terms of actual addiction, the number of young people in the UK receiving help levelled off in 2009–2010 after rising steadily in the previous decade (NTA, 2010). This was not necessarily an indication that more young people were 'using' and becoming 'dependent' on drugs, however, but was maybe due to an improvement in the identification of young drug users and better signposting to services and support. We look at some treatment practices aimed at young people below.

'Legal highs'

A relatively new phenomenon is the increasing use of so-called legal highs. These are substances that act as stimulants, alter or enhance mood, but which contain no substances deemed illegal. They are mainly sold via the internet, and their use is an increasing trend across Europe. Recent surveys show a higher rate of use in the UK than in any other country in the European Union, and according to the UNODC Report (2013) a total of 670,000 people aged 15 to 24 have experimented with these substances.

'Legal highs' are relatively new and there is evidence that young people in the UK are taking them rather than, or as well as, other substances. The health impacts are hard to pin down as yet, although there have been deaths linked to their use (NPSAD, 2013). Currently, the manufacturers and internet distributors of these substances are engaged in something of a game of 'cat and mouse' with legislators and politicians, with pressure growing from the public for more decisive action. The UK government is currently considering a blanket ban of all such substances sold on the internet.

Signs and symptoms of substance use/misuse

Anyone working with young people, whether in a formal setting such as a school, college or university, or in an informal setting such as a youth or sports club, needs to be able to recognize the signs of substance use/misuse. The signs and symptoms listed below are by no means always associated with substance use/misuse but are an indication that further investigation is required to establish that it is not the cause.

- Marked and uncharacteristic mood swings, aggressive or apathetic behaviour;

- Truancy and/or lateness for school/college/university or work;
- Deterioration in personal hygiene and dress;
- Sudden and marked change of habits, a loss of purpose in life, lacking motivation or personal goal;
- Unusual conflict with authority figures;
- Short-term memory loss and deterioration in performance, loss of concentration and/or loss of coordination;
- Poor appetite and weight loss or eating binges;
- Excessive borrowing of money. Stealing from family and/or friends;
- Selling of personal belongings;
- Use of drug slang and references;
- Frequent short visits from new or older friends/short excursions from home;
- Suffering a succession of colds and episodes of illnesses such as flu which persist for an unusually long time;
- Depression, shyness and poor self-image;
- Spending time away from home, especially overnight;
- Excessive sleeping, usually after time away from home;
- 'Drunken' behaviour, slurred speech.

The problem, as parents of many adolescents will tell you, is that many of these signs and symptoms are characteristic of 'normal' adolescent behaviour too! Nevertheless, they constitute a helpful checklist for professionals working with young people. Other signs to look out for would be the actual physical evidence of possible drug use:

- Cigarette lighters, matches (especially if a non-smoker);
- Knives, metal foil, drink can and bottle tops discoloured by heat;
- Clay, wooden, glass or ceramic long-stemmed pipes (chillums);
- Home-made 'hubble bubble' pipes (bongs) or other similar devices;
- Large cigarette papers, short cardboard tubes (roaches);
- Cigarette filters and cotton wool;
- Spoons discoloured by heat, often with a bent stem;

- Lemon juice, vinegar, ascorbic and citric acid;
- Tourniquets, syringes, needles, swabs and water ampoules;
- The use of strongly scented products to disguise smell of other substance use.

Theories of motivation for substance use/misuse

At the beginning of this chapter we asked why it is that some young people use and/or misuse substances. The importance of understanding a young person's motivation to use or misuse substances is that, hopefully, we can identify important risk and protective factors and use this knowledge to design interventions and educational responses to minimize risk and reduce harm.

Genetic theories

These suggest that an individual's genetic makeup predisposes them towards the likelihood of substance use/misuse. The main evidence lies in the way patterns of use and addiction can run in families. Schuckit (1980) developed the genetic predisposition theory, but also acknowledged that other factors – such as the availability of the substance – must be present too. A purely genetic explanation is almost impossible to prove in reality as there are so many other possible influences, or 'confounding variables', that could act upon a young person (Innovation with Substance and Southampton Healthy Schools, 2011).

Psychopharmacology theories

Psychopharmacological theories deal with substance abuse, addiction and treatment by focusing on the chemical reactions induced by drug use. Addiction can be explained, for example, in the 'incentive-sensitization' theory, which suggests that addictive behaviour is caused by the drug-induced changes – feelings/sensitization – in the nervous system (Innovation with Substance and Southampton Healthy Schools, 2011). Biological factors are particularly significant when responding to the needs of young people experiencing addiction. They underpin medical responses such as substituting less harmful substances (such as methadone) for more harmful ones (such as heroin) as part of a behavioural 'weaning' process, culminating ultimately in the cessation of all substance use. It is recognized, however, that substance use has psychological dimensions which also need to be addressed.

Psychological theories

Reinforcement theory is based on the idea central to behaviourism that individuals will tend to maximize positive experiences and minimize negative ones, and will pursue or avoid specific behaviours in accordance with past experiences. Reinforcement can be 'positive' – the increase of pleasure – or 'negative' – the cessation of stress, discomfort or pain. These types of reinforcement can develop in such a way that, initially, it is positive reinforcement that takes place, followed by addiction and then negative reinforcement in continued substance use. This theory has proved to be popular but does not explain variations in reactions between individuals – not everyone who uses drugs becomes addicted (Innovation with Substance and Southampton Healthy Schools, 2011).

There are several psychological explanations grouped under the category of 'personality theories'. All tend towards a social psychological explanation. One example is the 'inadequate personality' or 'deviant personality' theory developed in the 1970s (Kaplan, 1975). The suggestion is that it is problems in the individual's emotional life such as poorly developed self-esteem, self-rejection and social rejection, which predisposes the individual to use drugs as a means to escape their reality. More recently it has been pointed out that substance users actually have more close friendships than non-users, and sociological theories appear to support this argument that individuals rarely begin substance use alone (Innovation with Substance and Southampton Healthy Schools, 2011).

Sociological theories

'Social control theory' has proved popular with those who point to the 'laissez faire' and 'liberalization' approach to parenting and schooling associated with the 1960s and 1970s. Hirschi (1969) first developed this theory, asserting that substance use is caused by an absence of the social controls that encourage conformity, and that if no such controls exist substance use occurs naturally. The key argument is that the more attached to conventional society a person is, the less likely they are to engage in behaviour which violates its values (Innovation with Substance and Southampton Healthy Schools, 2011).

'Self-control theory' has its roots in research into the causes of criminal behaviour (Hirschi and Gottfredson, 1990). It builds on social control theory in that it shares the assumption that crime, including drug use, is natural and would always happen in the absence of controls. The crux of the theory is that people who engage in behaviours such as drug taking, without regard for the social and legal consequences, lack self-control, caused, they argue, by a lack of parental socialization. This theory also shares many of its key assumptions with 'Social Disorganization theory' which argues that substance use occurs where communities and families are unable, or unwilling, to take responsibility for controlling deviant behaviour. As a result, these behaviours flourish and create the perfect environment for continued substance use. These theories often seem to ignore the fact that many forms of substance use – alcohol in particular – are actually passed down the generations as part of familial and social conventions, and that this most often happens without harmful effects.

'Social Learning theory' was originally developed by Sutherland (1939), and suggests that crime and deviance are often learned in close relationships. The key mechanism for it to flourish is an association with social contacts who define crime and deviance in favourable terms, as okay and as 'normal'.

'Subcultural theory', also known as 'selective interaction' or the 'socialization model', was first proposed in the 1950s by Becker (cited in Goode, 2011). Subcultural theory suggests that it is involvement in specific groups or social circles that matters. This contradicts the traditional view that motivation to use substances precedes actual substance use, arguing instead that individuals first use substances in a social context and then go on to develop further motives to continue using them. Here, it is the engagement with the subculture that is the key factor in determining substance use (Innovation with Substance and Southampton Healthy Schools, 2011). In the context of working with young people this has particular significance in relation to 'peer-pressure' influence.

'Primary socialization theory' argues that normative and deviant behaviours are 'learned' and that norms for social behaviours, including substance use, are learned mainly in the home and at school. Weak bonds with family and school increase the chances that young people will go on to bond with deviant peer groups that engage in behaviours such as substance use (Oetting et al., 1998). 'Conflict theory' builds on primary socialization theory, but takes a wider view, embracing social and economic structures and conditions. It focuses specifically on heavy, chronic use of 'hard' drugs, arguing that this behaviour is often linked to social class and inequalities of opportunity (Innovation with Substance and Southampton Healthy Schools, 2011).

'Gateway theories' are very much part of the current debate around young people's substance use (Degenhardt et al., 2010). The central argument is that a 'gateway' drug such as cannabis causes users to be at increased risk of using other 'harder' drugs. Supporters of this theory assert that the use of 'soft' drugs can create a need for further, stronger experiences. This 'need' can be either physiological or psychological. For example, if use of a 'soft' drug appears to have no negative effects, it undermines the negative reputation surrounding all drugs, and thus renders advice against 'hard' drugs less persuasive. Also, some young people will be at increased risk of engaging in 'hard drug' use because of some of the reasons related to the other theories – peer pressure, for example. This all conspires to encourage 'graduation' to harder drugs. It has been argued that contact with 'soft' drugs increases the chances also of coming into contact with 'hard' drug suppliers. However, the actual link between so-called gateway drugs and use of 'hard drugs' appears to be weak (Putney, 2002).

Not all 'gateways' are into illegal substance use, however. Recent psychological research has begun to explore how patterns of alcohol use have changed in line with the rise of consumerism in recent decades. Researchers such as Pheonix (2005) have looked at the psychosocial impact of consumerism on adolescence, and highlight its significance in reshaping the context in which young people live. One feature of this has been the proactive marketing of alcohol to young people as part of a desirable, high status lifestyle by the drinks industry. Much of this marketing has an effect which operates in direct contradiction to those messages advocated by health promotion organizations. Leyshon (2011), for example, has highlighted the risks associated with internet-based marketing of alcohol to young people. This is an area of research which needs further development as part of the 'honest discussion' advocated by Sigman (2011) mentioned earlier.

In summary, we can say that substance use depends on a wide ranging and complex interaction of personal, cultural and environmental factors which all need to be considered. Most theorists claim that the factors they explore are part of a bigger picture. Overall, an understanding of risk and protective factors gives us the best opportunity to understand the reasons behind young people's drug use.

Risk and protective factors

A Home Office-sponsored systematic review of studies of risk factors was conducted by Frisher et al. (2007). It defined risk factors as:

> ...an individual attribute, individual characteristic, situational condition, or environmental context that increases the probability of drug use or abuse or a transition in level of involvement in drugs. (Home Office, 2007, p. 3)

The review highlighted the following factors:

Personal (biological or psychological) – that are 'given' and cannot be changed

- Genetic predisposition
- Gender
- Age
- Ethnicity

- Life-events
- Mental illness or depression
- Hedonism (pleasure/sensation seeking)

Personal (behavioural or attitudinal) – factors that can be changed by policy or lifestyle changes

- Anti-social behaviour
- Law breaking (delinquency)
- Early onset of smoking
- Early onset of alcohol use
- Attitude towards substance use
- Alienation/disaffection to school and society generally
- Low religiosity
- Dealing with drugs

Personal (interpersonal relationships) – relationships with friends and family

- Poor family relationships – lack of bonding
- Parental management – lack of parental control/lack of mutual respect
- Family conflict
- Peer group in trouble or using drugs
- Poor social support networks

Structural (environmental and economic) – including issues outside of the individual's control

- Socioeconomic status – poverty
- Schooling
- Neighbourhood disorder

- Lack of local opportunities both for leisure and employment

- Availability of drugs

It is not enough to simply see one protective factor outweighing one risk factor as they do not all carry equal weight. We can conclude, however, that by maximizing protective factors and minimizing risk factors we will be more successful in guiding young people away from harmful substance use. Harm reduction and risk minimization is the main approach adopted currently in the UK, referring to a range of interventions designed to reduce the harmful consequences associated with substance use. It accepts that the use of substances is an inevitable feature of the human experience, and recognizes that containment and reduction of harm is a more feasible approach than efforts to eliminate substance use altogether. We will now review some of the major treatments and responses designed to reduce harm and minimize risk related to substance use by young people.

Treatments and responses

Education around substance use/misuse

As with all health issues, schools are a major site for health education approaches to substance use. Curriculum time is limited, however, and it is vital that time is used well, focusing on the substances most relevant to young people. As we have seen, relatively few young people will find themselves in contact with Class A drugs such as heroin, whereas a high percentage will find themselves in contact with alcohol, tobacco, cannabis and volatile substances. This suggests that we need to focus on providing young people with an understanding of what they could be facing well before they are confronted with them in social situations. Just as importantly, we also need to equip them with skills and strategies to help them respond with informed decisions.

The Drug Education Forum (DEF) is a valuable source of information and guidance for those working with young people in the school setting and in informal settings. Central to the DEF's mission is the belief that:

> ...drug education should help children and young people develop their knowledge about drugs, their skills in taking decisions, and to develop a positive attitude towards their own health.

They argue that drug education should not be the sole responsibility of schools but of the whole community, including parents, teachers, health professionals, the media and government.

Key characteristics of effective substance use/misuse education programmes

The DEF recommends that drug education programmes have the following characteristics:

- Active teaching and learning strategies
- A broad skills base – not just knowledge
- The teacher as a facilitator – not didactic teaching
- A well-trained, confident, competent and supported workforce to deliver drug education
- Curriculum time to commit to drug education – no quick fixes, part of planned programme of PSHE
- Planned to meet the needs of young people taking into account local data, risk and protective factors and listening to what the young people say they want out of their drug education.

These findings support the guidance provided to schools in NICE public health guidance 23 (2010). For example, they recommend that smoking prevention interventions should be:

- fun, engaging, factual, interactive and age appropriate;
- include strategies for resisting the pressure to smoke;
- part of the wider PSHE curriculum prior to secondary school.

Education strategies should also aim to develop decision-making skills through active teaching and learning techniques, including strategies for enhancing self-esteem and resisting the pressure to smoke from family, peers, the media and the tobacco industry.

Web-assisted interventions

Active teaching and learning techniques are recommended by bodies such as the PSHE Association, NICE and other health education bodies and there are an increasing number of internet and web-assisted intervention programmes for tackling risk-taking behaviours. There is, as yet, little in the way of academic evaluation of such interventions, but NICE (2013) suggests that the evidence available to date indicates that web-based programmes could be useful for some children and young people in preventing smoking. They suggest they are best used as an additional tool alongside other forms of adult-led interventions, rather than as replacements for them. Further evaluative research to assess their impact is needed.

Peer-led interventions

In the last decade there has been a concerted effort by policy makers, senior leaders in schools and practitioners working with children and young people to ensure that the voice of children and young people is central to the planning, resourcing, delivery and evaluation of health education programmes. There has been an increase in the number of interventions that are planned and delivered by young people themselves, including smoking prevention/cessation pro- grammes, and peer-led programmes are seen by many as the way forward in addressing risk-taking behaviour in young people (Starkey et al., 2009).

The Cycle of Change

The 'stages of change' model developed by Prochasaka and DiClements (1982) has been an important influence on treatment services in the UK. Initially devised to describe the process people go through to give up smoking, it has been seen as applicable to other forms of substance misuse and problem behaviour too (see Figure 9.1).

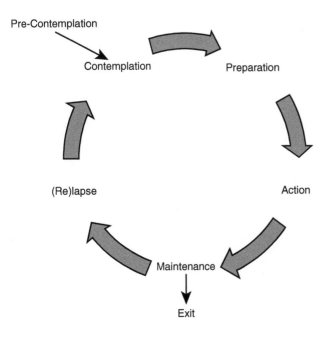

Stage of Change	Characteristics	Techniques
Pre-Contemplation	Not currently considering change: 'Ignorance is bliss'. The person does not acknowledge a problem exists.	Validate lack of readiness Clarify: decision is theirs Encourage reevaluation of current behaviour Encourage self-exploration, not action Explain and personalize the risk
Contemplation	Ambivalent about change: 'Sitting on the fence' Not considering change within the next month	Validate lack of readiness Clarify: decision is theirs Encourage evaluation of pros and cons of behaviour change Identify and promote new, positive outcome expectations
Preparation	Some experience with change and are trying to change: 'Testing the waters' Planning to act within 1 month	Identify and assist in problem solving re: obstacles. Help client identify social support Verify that client has underlying skills for behaviour change Encourage small initial steps
Action	Practicing new behaviour for 3–6 months. The decision to change can be all consuming.	Focus on restructuring cues and social support Bolster self-efficacy for dealing with obstacles Combat feelings of loss and reiterate long-term benefits
Maintenance	Continued commitment to sustaining new behaviour Post-6 months to 5 years. The change has been integrated into the person's life. Some support may still be needed. When we are able to maintain what we have achieved we exit the cycle.	Plan for follow-up support Reinforce internal rewards Discuss coping with relapse
Lapse	A temporary return to 'old' behaviours and unhelpful thoughts, feelings and behaviours	Avoid judgement. Support and discuss where they are on the cycle of change. Explore factors that triggered lapse. Reevaluate their readiness to change.
Relapse	Resumption of old behaviours: 'Fall from grace'. Lapses and relapses are not viewed as 'failures'. It is accepted that change is difficult. When relapse occurs, several journeys through the cycle may be necessary to make last changes. Each time the person is encouraged to review, reflect and learn from the experience.	Evaluate trigger for relapse Reassess motivation and barriers Plan stronger coping strategies

Figure 9.1 The Cycle of Change

An important emphasis in treatment programmes is that they should be 'client focused'. Behaviour change requires practitioners to have appropriate skills, and, in particular, good listening skills and an understanding of the client-centred working model. It is important to stress that the 'cycle of change' model is not a treatment model but a way of looking at how people may feel about their substance use, and thus a way of exploring what type of intervention would be useful to them. We will now look at some interventions.

A solution-focused approach

The predominant approach to working with young people who use substances currently is the 'solution-focused approach'. The individual young person is placed at the centre of this type of intervention, and an emphasis is placed on establishing mutual respect and trust, building on the young person's own strengths and qualities. The approach is 'future orientated' and works within the young person's own frame of reference to achieve their chosen goals. A 'solution-focused approach' does not imply that there is always a solution to every life problem, but instead offers ways in which young people can be empowered to manage their problems better (O'Connell, 2003).

The philosophy implies a minimal intervention in the young person's life, and the therapeutic task is seen as raising the young person's awareness of constructive solutions that they already use in their lives and building upon these. The principle can be represented in these simple mantras:

- Small changes can lead to bigger changes
- If it ain't broke, don't fix it
- If it's working keep doing it
- If it's not working stop doing it
- Keep therapy as simple as possible.

Motivational Interviewing

Motivational Interviewing (MI) is more a way of being with people rather than a technique. It is intentionally directive in that it is focused on the resolution of ambivalence and moving the young person towards positive change. MI uses open questions to affirm, reflect and summarize. There are four underpinning principles to the approach:

1 *Express empathy* – Acceptance facilitates change. Blaming, criticism and judging have no place. Skilful reflective listening is fundamental. Ambivalence is normal.

2 *Developing discrepancy* – The young person rather than the professional should present the arguments for change. Change is motivated by a perceived discrepancy between present behaviour and important personal goals or values.

3 *Roll with resistance* – Avoid arguing for change. Any resistance is not directly opposed. Invite but do not impose new perspectives. The young person is the primary source in finding answers and solutions. Resistance is a signal to respond differently.

4 *Support self-efficacy* – An individual's belief in the possibility of change is an important motivator. It is the young person who is responsible for choosing and carrying out change. The professional's own belief in the young person's ability to change then becomes a self-fulfilling prophecy (Dixey, 2013).

Brief Interventions

Brief Interventions (BI) have been successfully used with different behaviours, including reducing alcohol use, and preventing drug use and driving. BIs are aimed at young people who may not as yet be experiencing major health problems, but who need to be convinced that they are behaving in a way that could become harmful to their health. BIs can also be used with young people who have expressed concern or requested advice about substance use but who are not experiencing dependency. BIs are usually referred to as 'opportunistic' in that a person has not complained about the problem with substance use, and is actually seeking help for other reasons. For example, a young person visits the GP because of a reoccurring chest complaint, which is used as an opportunity for a BI in smoking cessation.

A BI has been defined as having five essential steps:

1 Screening/assessment of substance use and feedback

2 Negotiation and agreement of goals for reducing substance use

3 Familiarization of the individual with behaviour modification techniques

4 Reinforcement with self-help materials

5 Follow-up telephone support or further visits

(Fleming and Manwell, 1999)

There is a growing body of evidence supporting the 'Brief Intervention' approach for adults (Moyer et al., 2002; Kaner et al., 2007). Higher risk and 'increasing risk drinkers' who receive brief advice are twice as likely to moderate their drinking 6 to12 months after an intervention when compared to drinkers receiving no intervention (Wilk et al., 1997). The effectiveness of this approach with young drinkers is not yet clear, however.

Specialist substance misuse services for young people

The majority of young people who use substances do so either on a recreational or experimental basis that is unlikely to become problematic. It is unlikely that they will need, or want, to be referred on to a specialist young person's substance misuse service. Nevertheless, they may well need information, advice and support around their use if any of the following applies:

- Their knowledge in relation to the substances they are using is low
- Their knowledge in relation to other substances is low
- Their knowledge in relation to the legal aspects of substance use is low
- They feel under pressure to use drugs.

A specialist professional working with young people may be involved in providing the following:

- Information and advice in relation to specific substances
- Key harm reduction messages such as not mixing substances, not using on your own and not using anything you cannot identify
- Developing self-esteem and life skills, such as strategies to resist peer pressure
- Facilitating access to other diversionary activities.

Screening tools

Various screening tools have been developed to support professionals working with young people. The assessment and screening for young people's substance misuse is important to ensure that they get the appropriate intervention to address their substance use issues. The National Treatment Agency of the NHS sets out a four-tiered approach to drug treatment for both adults and young people, which, despite a considerable reduction in local authority funding in recent years, continues to provide a framework for an integrated and comprehensive children and young people's service.

The Four-Tiered Framework

- **Tier 1 ...** Ensures universal access and continuity of care to all young people. In addition, it aims to identify and screen those who may be vulnerable to substance misuse and identify those with difficulties in relation to existing substance use. It will be concerned with education improvement, prevention, maintenance of health, educational attainment and identification of risks or child protection issues. It will also engage in embedding advice and information concerning substances, within a general health improvement agenda. These should be seen as mainstream services for young people and could involve a variety of agencies and agents including teachers, school nurses, youth workers, community workers, health visitors and GPs.

- **Tier 2 ...** Youth-orientated services, offered by practitioners with some drug and alcohol experience and youth-work specialist knowledge, should be working at this level. The aim and purpose of this tier is to be concerned with reduction of risks and vulnerabilities, reintegration and maintenance of young people in mainstream services.

- **Tier 3 is ...** For young people with more complex needs. Young people's specialist drug services and other specialized services, which work with complex cases requiring multidisciplinary team-based work, should be working at this level. The aim of Tier 3 services is to deal with complex and often multiple needs of children or young people and not just with the particular substance problems. Tier 3 services also work towards reintegrating and including the child/young person in their family, community, school or place of work.

- **Tier 4 is ...** Provision of highly specialized forms of intervention for young drug users with complex care needs. It is recognized that, for a very small number of people, there is a need for intensive interventions, which could include short-term substitute prescribing, detoxification and respite care away from home. Respite care away might be offered in a number of different ways, such as residential units, enhanced fostering and supported hostels. The success of this tier depends very much on the multi-agency approach. All professionals working with these young people have a contribution to make in order to meet the requirements of the National Drug Strategy and key performance indicators set by government.

(NTA/NHS, 2005)

For the majority of young people Tier 1 and Tier 2 levels of support are what is required. A Tier 3 referral is required if one or more of the following is identified:

- The young person is 13 years of age or younger and taking substances

- If the substance is being used to block out thoughts and/or feelings, or to cope with certain situations they find difficult

- The young person is pregnant and using substances

- The young person is injecting or requesting injecting advice

- The young person is using large enough quantities of a substance that they could overdose; i.e. alcohol, heroin or using substances they cannot identify

- The young person is mixing substances such as alcohol, heroin, methadone and benzodiazepines

- The young person is financing their use in ways that increase their vulnerability, e.g. engaging in increasingly offending behaviour or being sexually exploited

- The use of drugs is causing significant problems in their life, i.e. mental health problems, physical complications from use, threat to personal safety or relationship breakdown

- The young person requires advice and information on pre- and post-test counselling on Hepatitis B and C and HIV

- The young person is disengaging from education because of their substance use

- The young person has been excluded from school related to substance use.

Referral pathways vary from area to area and professionals working with young people need to familiarize themselves with their own local service structures (NHS/NTA, 2005).

Conclusions

This chapter has attempted to give an overview of the issues surrounding young people and substance use in the UK. Whilst substance use among young people is a concern we must remember that:

- The majority of young people will never use an illegal drug.

- Many will, at some stage in their transition from childhood to adulthood, be occasional users of substances, particularly alcohol and tobacco.

We have seen in this chapter that there are complex motivating factors behind young people's use of substances, whether legal or illegal. We have explored briefly the idea that adolescents are more likely than other age groups to take risks, and that some substance use may be an almost inevitable rite of passage for many young people. But what we have also learnt is that most young people will not go on to be problem drug users. What is undeniable, however, is that all children and young people will be exposed to the effects of substance use in the communities where they live, and it is therefore paramount that professionals and parents alike are supported to respond appropriately.

Suggested Further Reading

Aggleton, P., Ball, A. and Mane, P. (eds) (2005) *Sex, Drugs and Young People: International Perspectives (Sexuality, Culture and Health)*. London: Routledge.

Crome, I. B., Hamid, G. and Gilvarry, E. (eds) (2004) *Young People and Substance Misuse*. London: Gaskell.

Department for Education and Skills (DfES) (2004) *Drugs: Guidance for Schools*. London: Crown Copyright.

Emmett, D. and Nice, G. (2006) *Understanding Street Drugs: A Handbook of Substance Misuse for Parents, Teachers and Other Professionals* (2nd edition). London: Jessica Kingsley Publishers.

Fletcher, A., Bonell, C., Sorhaindo, A. and Strange, V. (2009) How might schools influence young people's drug use? Development of theory from qualitative case-study research. *Journal of Adolescent Health [serial online]*. 45 (2), 126–132. Available from: Child Development & Adolescent Studies, Ipswich, MA. Accessed 21 October 2015.

Sunstein, C. R. (2008). Adolescent risk-taking and social meaning: A commentary. *Developmental Review*. 28, 145–152.

10

PROMOTING HEALTH AND WELL-BEING IN YOUNG PEOPLE: CHANGING YOUNG PEOPLE, OR CHANGING SOCIETY?

> We need to stop thinking of spend on healthcare for children and young people and instead think of investing in the health of children and young people as a route to improving the economic health of our nation. (Dame Sally Davies, Chief Medical Officer, 2012)

In 2010, the formation of a Coalition government, after an indecisive general election, marked the beginning of the so-called austerity agenda. This involved significantly cutting public spending as a means of reducing the fiscal deficit generated by the last New Labour governments' 'bail-out' of failing banks in 2008. This agenda has had a significant impact on programmes aimed at promoting the health and well-being of young people. One of its most immediate casualties was the burgeoning Youth Work sector, which, on the back of New Labour's 'Every Child Matters' (2003) agenda, was on the point of becoming formalized into a fully professionalized area of work, with distinct training programmes and career paths. Those plans were swiftly shelved, and many local authority youth work services have been severely reduced or dismantled altogether since then. The State has now effectively pulled out of Youth Work. Similarly, the National Healthy Schools programme was cut, and sweeping changes to the way schools are organized, governed and inspected, alongside changes to the curriculum, mean that schools find it increasingly difficult to remain as committed as before to health promotion activities.

NHS provision for young people has also been cut. 'Young Minds' (2014) reported that 34 out of 51 CAMHs departments have seen their budgets reduced since 2010. Hagell and Coleman (2015) state that real concern is emerging about the impact of these cuts, both to immediate levels of support provided to young people in need, and to the future health and well-being of the wider population of young people, who will grow into adults, carrying their health issues, problems, vulnerabilities – and costs – with them.

Health promotion for young people – Where are we headed?

Writing in the 1990s, the leading American researcher in childhood health Melvin Konner pointed out that:

> Psychology and biology alike predict that we will be preoccupied with ourselves and our own children, but their future and ours may hinge on how well we can transcend those preoccupations – on how much, in effect, we can care about other people's children. It may help to notice that other people's children will constitute the environment in which our children will spend most of their lives, our grandchildren grow up, and we ourselves spend our declining years. If they are healthy, educated and optimistic about their future, they will create one kind of environment; if they are sick, ignorant and enraged, another. (Konner, 1991, p. 411)

That warning proved prophetic. The mass of epidemiological and social data gathered and analysed by Wilkinson and Pickett (2010) and Dorling (2013) amongst others illustrates how the United States has become a significant 'negative outlier' among affluent countries, with epidemic proportions of physical and mental ill health, teenage pregnancy rates, drug and alcohol problems, violent crime and poor educational performance – all disproportionately affecting poor, and particularly black, young Americans.

The bleakness of this situation stands in stark contrast to countries such as Japan, Sweden, Norway, Denmark, Finland and the Netherlands, where levels of inequality are considerably less than those tolerated in the US, and where there is a great deal more commitment across the political spectrum to creating safe and supportive environments for children and young people to grow up in (Wilkinson and Pickett, 2010; James, 2007). This is not to say that the United States has no examples of good practice and policy to follow; or that the Scandinavian and northern Europeans have got it 'just right' – far from it. We would argue, however, that an evidence-based approach surely requires we look to follow examples with the best outcomes.

'Austerity' or 'Ideology'?

The current UK government argues that the 'austerity agenda' is a necessity, forced upon us by the 2008 economic crisis. This agenda can also be seen, however, as consistent with a longer term political trend in the UK, one followed by successive recent governments, and associated with the dominance of a so-called neoliberal economic ideology. This ideology advocates government withdrawal from active intervention in people's lives, leaving them to make their own choices in the free market of commerce, ideas and lifestyles. In line with this approach the current government has increasingly pushed responsibility for addressing young people's health and well-being back onto families and individuals, steering policy away from strategies involving state intervention and/or the regulation of corporate behaviour.

In an era when corporate power and influence over young people's health and well-being has never been greater this is, we would argue, naive at best, and, at worst, amounts to neglect; allowing corporate interests to pursue marketing strategies known to be detrimental to the health and well-being of children and young people. One of the main themes to emerge as we have looked at the various issues identified in this book is the pervasive influence of commercial interests – particularly the food, fashion, music, information technology and marketing industries – in targeting young people in ways that too often undermine their health and well-being.

Recent governments in the UK – New Labour, Coalition and Conservative alike – have shown great reluctance, for example, to challenge the powerful food industry lobby, and have instead opted for a so-called nudge approach, which argues that if people are provided with enough information about the benefits of healthy eating and taking more exercise then they are able to make healthy choices for themselves. This approach has been challenged by Dorling (2014), however, who describes it as 'giving the poor marketing instead of decent food' (p. 136). He argues that it is based on 'a pernicious and persistent myth' that the reason poor people eat badly is because they make bad choices rather than that they are unable to afford a healthier diet. We would add that it also ignores the extent to which positive health promotion messages are swamped beneath a deluge of product and brand promotion messages pouring from the powerful marketing machines of the food industry.

Corporate advertising and marketing campaigns are often designed specifically to persuade children and young people that possessing their products, or using their 'brand', is one of the hallmarks of a successful, popular, 'high-status' individual. The amount of money directed at these campaigns suggests that they produce high returns in promoting 'market share', 'brand loyalty' and increased profits – in other words, they work! Discussion around 'risk' in adolescence often seems to ignore marketing influence, however, and sees it as a problem of individuals making poor decisions, rather than vulnerable young people responding to powerful psychological cues to which they are particularly susceptible. Advertisers are well aware of how to 'get to' young people, as shown by the massive profitability of social networking sites, driven primarily by their use to corporate marketing.

Health promotion strategies, such as those aimed at reducing obesity for instance, often involve targeting communities identified as especially vulnerable, such as poor and ethnic minority communities, school age children, and individuals and families identified as 'high risk'. Such an approach may have some justification, but arguably far more could be achieved, both in terms of health and well-being, and effective use of resources, by more active government intervention aimed at countering the promotion of an 'obesogenic environment'. For example:

- Banning fast food advertising aimed at children below the age of 10.

- Stricter control and regulation of what goes into 'fast' and retailed food, in recognition that much of what is currently used is poor quality and sometimes actually harmful.

- Much clearer labelling of the levels of fat and sugar content in food products.

- The active promotion of healthier and more diverse modes of food production and consumption – including encouraging a greater diversity of producers and retailers.

- Taxing food products high in sugar and other harmful substances – the so-called sugar tax.

These suggestions may seem rather grandiose, but they are all policies that have been successfully pursued by governments elsewhere – Sweden, France, Finland, Greece – who have committed themselves to actively using public policy to promote the health and well-being of children and young people. And a sugar tax was one of the main recommendations of a recent report to the government on reducing sugar consumption by Public Health England (2015).

If a further example of a highly successful 'big' policy approach to health promotion of this kind were needed then we would point to the remarkable sea-change in attitudes to smoking, driven by a direct 'interventionist' approach by governments across the developed world – including the UK – to regulate both the actual activity of smoking and, critically, the selling and marketing of tobacco products. The beneficial effects of this approach have now begun to show in declining rates of smoking-related disease in the UK, and with them the high costs of treatments.

The smoking example shows what can be achieved by public health policy which directly challenges commercial interests when they promote substances and behaviours known to be harmful to health and well-being. Whilst we don't advocate the micro-management of people's behaviour by government, nor argue that all corporate behaviour is as irresponsible as that of the tobacco industry, we would argue that protecting young people from commercial interests where these clearly promote unhealthy life choices is on a par with protecting them from pernicious individuals who would abuse and exploit them.

Limits of The Big Society?

Another approach often advocated as an alternative to direct state intervention is the 'self-help' model. This model has drawn support from across the political spectrum in the UK as a way of building and providing community-based public services – and Prime Minister David Cameron has made it something of a personal crusade through the so-called Big Society project. There is widespread recognition that such projects, if soundly funded, well planned, based on sound, evidence-based knowledge and practice, and locally based, can help to empower local communities and individuals. For these reasons a 'self-help' model, drawing on the long-established traditions of the voluntary sector, and enhanced by diverse social-entrepreneurial models, can add to and enhance the quality of community-based support systems.

Such models also have their limitations, however. Projects are often reliant on small, vulnerable funding streams and local authority contracts that are renewed yearly. This means they are often unable to either pay well or provide long-term job security, and thus have a workforce that is often transitory; trends that are becoming more acute as central government continues to impose major cuts on local government budgets. There also lurks a suspicion that the 'Big Society' project is designed to plug gaps left by cuts to public services – a way of doing things cheaply rather than effectively.

Experience elsewhere, including the US, has shown that the best and most effective 'self-help' models are those supported by secure, usually national or local government funding streams. Konner (1991) illustrated this in relation to the much lauded 'head start' programme as it was rolled out to more and more areas, but with diminishing levels of federal government funding. This not only led to a decline in the quality of the service being provided, but also in the cost benefits that had been one of the main arguments underpinning the setting up of the programme in the first place, leading Konner to angrily retort that:

> Somebody in accounting should go over the figures with the leaders of our government, since it is plain that our failure to fund Head Start more fully is fiscal irresponsibility. (Konner, 1991, p. 418)

There are strong echoes here in the current situation in the UK, where the 'Sure Start' programme, using 'Head Start' as a model, has been cut back in many areas – a policy which may well have future auditors of public finances scratching their head when long-term cost/benefit analyses are worked out.

Conclusions

The overall picture of young people's health in the UK today is something of a paradox. It can reasonably be argued that, in terms of physical health, current generations of young people are among the healthiest ever. In previous chapters we have focused on a number of known threats that need to be monitored and addressed, including issues around sexual health, nutrition, alcohol and substance abuse. Despite this, however, it is recognized that young people generally are, physically at least, the healthiest of all age groups in society.

When it comes to mental and emotional health, however, the picture is much more worrying. We appear to be witnessing an epidemic of mental and emotional health problems in young people. The reasons undoubtedly lie in growing up and living in an increasingly pressured psychological environment as educational, technological, marketing and economic factors all bear down on them as they strive to negotiate the environment adults have created for them. The greatest current threat to the health, happiness and well-being of young people is, without question, the failure of our political and economic elites to tackle those issues, and to pursue a policy agenda more likely to exacerbate, rather than eradicate, health inequalities. This is especially frustrating given that so much is known about how to address the issues we have discussed in this book.

Hagell and Coleman (2014) state optimistically that young people's health and well-being appears to be moving up the political agenda. The recommendations of the 'Improving Young People's Health and Wellbeing Framework' (PHE/AYPH, 2014) centre on six principles:

1 Putting relationships at the centre

2 Focusing on what helps young people feel well and able to cope

3 Reducing health inequalities

4 Championing integrated services

5 Understanding changing health needs as young people develop

6 Delivering accessible, youth friendly services.

These principles, it is hoped, will set the agenda for health promotion for young people in the UK in the immediate future. They will only succeed, however, if the political will exists to see health promotion as one of the most important investments a country can make in its young people's, and by definition its own, future. As Roberts (2012) puts it:

> Having the evidence is only part of the picture. Having the political will and the combination of knowledge and skills to implement programmes or interventions which reduce inequalities is key to creating fair shares in child health. (p. 2)

The ongoing debate around such issues is a critical part of the process by which citizens and communities can strive to gain greater control over the environment in which their children and young people live, learn and grow, from those whose interests are primarily commercial and/or ideological in nature. One of the greatest achievements of the post-Second World War generation in the UK was the health-promoting transformation of the environment in which children and young people lived and grew up. We are all the beneficiaries of that transformation. The struggle now is to ensure that our legacy is as positive for the generations growing up in our care.

Suggested Further Reading

CSDH (2008) *Closing the Gap in a Generation: Health Equity through Action on the Social Determinants of Health.* Final Report of the Commission on the Social Determinants of Health. Geneva: World Health Organization.

Davies, S. (2013) *Annual Report of the Chief Medical Officer 2013: Our Children Deserve Better.* London: HMSO.

Dorling, D. (2013) *Unequal Health: The Scandal of Our Times.* London: Policy Press.

Hagell, A. and Coleman, J. (2014) *Young People's Health: Update 2014.* London: Association for Young People's Health (AYPH).

Public Health England/AYPH (2014) *Improving Young People's Health: A Framework for Public Health.* London: PHE/AYPH.

Roberts, H. (2012) *What Works in Reducing Inequalities in Child Health* (2nd edition). Bristol: Policy Press.

Wilkinson, R. and Pickett, K. (2010) *The Spirit Level: Why Equality Is Better for Everyone.* London: Penguin.

REFERENCES

Akabas, S., Lederman, S. and Moore, B. (2012) *Textbook of Obesity: Biological, Psychological and Cultural Influences.* Oxford: Wiley/Blackwell.

American Psychiatric Association (2013) Diagnostic and Statistical Manual of the American Psychiatric Association Edition 5. Arlington, VA: American Psychiatric Association Publishing.

Arai, L. (2009) *Teenage Pregnancy: The Making and Unmaking of a Problem*: Bristol: Policy Press.

Armstrong, T. (2010) *The Power of Neurodiversity: Unleashing the Advantages of Your Differently Wired Brain.* Philadelphia: Da Capo Books.

Atlantic (1998) Neurodiversity. http://www.theatlantic.com/magazine/archive/1998/09/neurodiversity/305909/ (Accessed 28/04/16).

Attwood, T. (2008) *The Complete Guide to Aspergers' Syndrome.* London: Jessica Kingsley.

Australian Geographic (2011) Animals Getting High: 10 Common Drunks. www.australiangeographic.com.au/topics/wildlife/2011/10/animals-getting-high-10-common-drunks (Accessed 23/03/14).

Bailey, S. and Shooter, M. (2009) *The Young Mind: An Essential Guide to Mental Health for Young Adults, Parents and Teachers.* London: Royal College of Psychiatrists.

Bainbridge, D. (2009) *Teenagers: A Natural History.* London: Portobello Books.

Barber, B. K. (2005) Parenting Support, Psychological Control, Behavioural Control: Assessing Relevance across Time, Culture and Method. *Monographs of the Society for Research in Child Development;* Vol. 70, No. 4. Oxford: Blackwell.

Barnes, C. and Oliver, M. (2012) *The New Politics of Disability.* Basingstoke: Palgrave Macmillan.

Barton J. and Pretty J. (2010) What is the best dose of nature and green exercise for mental health? A meta-study analysis. *Environmental Science & Technology.* DOI 10.1021/es903183r.

BBC News (27 May 2011) Alcohol-related hospital admissions reach record level. www.bbc.co.uk/news/health-13559455 (Accessed 18/03/14).

BBC News (2014) Teenage pregnancy rates lowest since 1969. www.bbc.co.uk/news/health-17190185 (Accessed 29/03/14).

Beresford, P. and Trevillion, S. (1995) *Developing Skills for Community Care: A Collaborative Approach.* London: Arena.

Biddle, L., Gunnell, D., Sharp, D. and Donovan, J. (2004) Factors influencing help seeking in mentally distressed young adults: A cross-sectional survey. *British Journal of General Practice.* 54, 248–253.

Blackburn, C., Read, J. and Spencer, N. (2012) Children with neurodevelopmental disabilities. In S. Davies C. Lemer (ed.), *Annual Report of the Chief Medical Officer 2012: Our Children Deserve Better.* London: HMSO.

Boland, P. (2008) British Drugs Policy: Problematising the distinction between legal and illegal drugs and the definition of the 'drugs problem'. *Probation Journal.* 55 (2), 171–187.

Bragg, S., Kehily, M. and Montgomery, H. (2013) Innocence..... In S. Bragg and M. Kehily (eds) *Children and Young People's Cultural Worlds.* Bristol: Policy Press.

Brook, Centre for HIV and Sexual Health, FPA (2009) *Young People and Pornography: A Briefing for Workers.* Leicester: The National Youth Agency.

Brown, F. J. (2005) ADHD and the philosophy of science. In C. Newnes, and N. Radcliffe (eds) *Making and Breaking Children's Lives.* Ross-on-Wye: PCCS Books, pp. 40–48.

Burthy, E. and Duffy, M. (2004) *Young People and Sexual Health.* Basingstoke: Palgrave Macmillan.

Burns, J. (2007) *The Descent of Madness: The Evolutionary Origins of Psychosis and the Social Brain.* London: Routledge.

Byron, T. (2008) *Safer Children in a Digital World: The Report of the Byron Review.* Nottingham: DCSF Publications.

Carnea, V. (2008) Does adventure education mitigate violent and aggressive behaviour in individuals and groups. *Countryside Recreational Network.* 16 (2),18–20.

Carr, N. (2010) *The Shallows: How the Internet Is Changing the Way We Think, Read and Remember.* London: Atlantic Books.

Carr, A. (2010) *Positive Psychology: The Science of Happiness and Human Strengths.* London: Routledge.

Channel 4 (2008) The Sex Education Show. www.channel4.com/programmes/the-sex-education-show/episode-guide/series-1/ (Accessed 10/01/14).

ChildLine (2008) Children talking to ChildLine about bullying. www.nspcc.org.uk (Accessed 28/04/16).

Coleman, J. (2007) Emotional health and well-being. In J. Coleman, L. B. Hendry and K. Kloep (eds) *Adolescence and Health.* Chichester: John Wiley & Sons, pp. 41–59.

Coleman, J. and Hagell, A. (eds) (2007) *Adolescence, Risk and Resilience: Against the Odds.* Chichester: John Wiley & Sons.

Coleman, J., Hendry, L. and Kloep, M. (2007) *Adolescence and Health.* Chichester: John Wiley & Sons.

Coleman, J. (2011) *The Nature of Adolescence* (4th edition). London: Routledge.

Contact a Family (2013) Contact a Family (CAF) Directory. www.cafamily.org.uk (Accessed 28/04/16).

CSDH (2008) Closing the Gap in a Generation: Health Equity through Action on the Social Determinants of Health. *Final Report of the Commission on the Social Determinants of Health.* Geneva: World Health Organization.

Daily Mail. (27 May 2011) Our binge-drinking nation: Alcohol-related hospital admissions double in a decade to top ONE MILLION a year. www.dailymail.co.uk/health/article-1391069/Alcohol-related-admissions-hospitals-tops-ONE-MILLION-year-time (Accessed 24/03/14).

Davies, C., Coleman, J. and Livingstone, S. (2014) *Digital Technologies in the Lives of Young People.* London: Routledge.

Degenhardt, L. et al. (2010) Evaluating the drug use 'gateway' theory using cross-national data: Consistency and associations of the order of initiation of drug use among participants in the WHO World Mental Health Surveys. *Drug and Alcohol Dependency.* 108 (1–2), 84–97.

DeGrandpre, R. (2000) *Ritalin Nation: Rapid-Fire Culture and the Transformation of Human Consciousness.* London: W.W. Norton & Company.

Dept for Children, Schools and Families and Dept of Health (2010) *Teenage Pregnancy Strategy: Beyond 2010.* London: HMSO.

Dept for Culture, Media and Sport (2007) *Taking Part: The National Survey of Culture, Leisure and Sport.* London: HMSO.

Dept for Education (2011) *Letting Children be Children: Report of the Independent Review of the Commercialisation and Sexualisation of Childhood. (The Bailey Review)* Norwich: TSO

Dept of Education (2003) *Every Child Matters.* London: HMSO.

Dept for Education and Skills (2004) *Drugs: Guidance for Schools.* London: HMSO.

Dept for Education and Skills (2006) *Teenage Pregnancy Next Steps: Guidance for Local Authorities & Primary Care Trusts on Effective Delivery of Local Strategies.* London: HMSO.

Dept for Employment and Education (2000) *Sex and Relationships Education Guidance.* London: HMSO.

Dept of Health (2011) *'You're Welcome': Quality Criteria for Young People Friendly Health Services.* London: HMSO.

Dept of Health (2013) *A Framework for Sexual Health Improvement in England.* London: HMSO.

Diamond, J. (1997) *Why Is Sex Fun? The Evolution of Human Sexuality.* New York: Basic Books.

Diamond, J. (2012) *The World Until Yesterday.* London: Penguin.

Dixey, R. (2013) *Health Promotion: Global Principles and Practice.* Oxford: CABI.

Dorling, D. (2011) *Injustice: Why Social Inequality Persists.* Bristol: Policy Press.

Dorling, D. (2014) *Inequality and the 1%.* London: Verso.

Duncan, S., Edwards, R. and Alexander, C. (2010) *Teenage Parenthood: What's the Problem?* London: Tufnell Press.

Dye, M., Green, S. and Bavalier, D. (2009) Increasing speed of processing with action video games. *Current Trends in Psychological Science.* 18 (6), 321–326.

Emmett, D. and Nice, G. (2006) *Understanding Street Drugs: A Handbook of Substance Misuse for Parents, Teachers and Other Professionals* (2nd edition). London: Jessica Kingsley Publishers.

Erikson, E. (1968) *Identity: Youth and Crisis.* New York: Norton.

Ewles, L. and Simnett, I. (2009) *Promoting Health: A Practical Guide.* London: Bailliere Tindall.

Family Planning Association (2011) *Sex & Relationships Education Factsheet.* London: FPA.

Fergusson, D. M. and Horwood, L. J. (2000) Does cannabis use encourage other forms of illicit drug use? *Addiction.* 95, 505–520.

Fergusson, D. M. and Horwood, L. J. (2003) Resilience to childhood adversity: results of a 21 year study. In S. Luthar (ed.) *Resilience and Vulnerability in the Context of Childhood.* Cambridge: Cambridge University Press, pp. 130–154.

Fisher, H. (2013) Mind the gap – pathways to psychosis. *The Psychologist.* 24 (11), 798–801.

Fleming, M. F. and Manwell, L. B. (1999) Brief intervention in primary care settings. a primary treatment method for at-risk, problem, and dependent drinkers. *Alcohol Research Health.* 23, 128–137.

Ford, J. (2005) *Right on Schedule: A Teen's Guide to Growth and Development.* Philadelphia: Mason Crest Publishers.

Frank Information for young people. www.talktofrank.com (Accessed 24/03/14).

Franklin, S. (2013) *Personalisation in Practice: Supporting Young People with Disabilities through the Transition to Adulthood.* London: Jessica Kingsley Publishers.

Frith, U. (2008) *Autism: A Very Short Introduction.* Oxford: Oxford University Press.

Gardener, H. (1983) *Frames of Mind: The Theory of Multiple Intelligences.* New York: Basic Books.

Gerhardt, S. (2010) *The Selfish Society: How We All Forgot to Love One Another and Made Money Instead.* London: Simon & Schuster.

Goode, E. (2006) The sociology of drug use. In C. D. Bryant and D. Peck (eds) *21st Century Sociology*, pp. 415–424.

Goode, E. (2011) *Drugs in American Society* (8th edition). New York: McGraw-Hill Education.

Goodley, D. (2013) Disability and psychology. In J. Swain, S. French, C. Barnes and C. Thomas (eds) *Disabling Barriers: Enabling Environments* (3rd edition). London: Sage, pp. 62–69.

Grandin, T. and Panek, R. (2014) *The Autistic Brain: Exploring the Strength of a Different Kind of Mind.* London: Rider.

Green, C. S. and Bevalier, D. (2006) Enumeration versus multiple object tracking: the case of action video games players. *Cognition.* 101, 217–245.

Greenfield, S. (2011) *ID: The Quest for Meaning in the 21st Century.* London: Sceptre.

Greenfield, S. (2014) *Mind Change: How Digital Technologies Are Leaving Their Mark on Our Brains.* London: Routledge.

Gross, R. (2010) *Psychology: The Science of Mind & Behaviour.* London: Hodder Arnold.

Hagell, A. (2012) *Changing Adolescence: Social Trends and Mental Health.* Bristol: Policy Press.

Hagell, A., Coleman, J. and Brooks, F. (2013) *Key Data on Adolescence 2013.* London: Association for Young People's Health.

Hagell, A. and Coleman, J. (2014) *Young People's Health: Update 2014.* London: Association for Young People's Health.

Hagell, A. and Rigby, E. (2014) *The Effectiveness of Prevention and Early Intervention to Promote Health Outcomes for Young People.* Paper prepared for Public Health England Annual Conference, 16/17 September 2014. Coventry: University of Warwick.

Harris, M. and Hall, E. L. (2014) *The Tree of Life Project with Young People with Diabetes.* AYPH Seminar Presentation. Child & Adolescent Diabetes Service. University College Hospital, London.

Hart, M. (1990) *Drumming at the Edge of Magic: A Journey into the Spirit of Percussion.* San Francisco: Harper.

Health Survey for England (2008) *Physical Activity and Fitness – Volume 1.* Leeds: The NHS Information Centre.

Hendrickx, S. (2010) *The Adolescent and Adult Neuro-diversity Handbook: Asperger Syndrome, ADHD, Dyslexia, Dyspraxia and Related Conditions.* London: Jessica Kingsley Publishers.

Hesmondhalgh, M. and Breakey, C. (2001) *Access and Inclusion for Children with Autistic Spectrum Disorders: 'Let Me In'.* London: Jessica Kingsley Publishers.

Hesse, R. and Williams, G. (1995) *Evolution and Healing: The New Science of Darwinian Medicine.* London: Weidenfeld & Nicolson.

Hewett, D., Firth, G., Barber, M. and Harrison, T. (2012) *The Intensive Interaction Handbook*. London: Sage.

Hobsbawm, E. (2014a) *The Age of Capital 1848-1875*. London: Abacus.

Hobsbawm, E. (2014b) *The Age of Empire 1875-1914*. London: Abacus.

Hollingworth, W. et al. (2012) Reducing smoking in adolescents: cost-effectiveness results from the cluster randomized ASSIST (A Stop Smoking In Schools Trial). *Nicotine & Tobacco Research.* 14 (2), 161–168.

Home Office (2007) *Predictive Factors for Illicit Drug Use among Young People: A Literature Review.* London: HMSO.

Home Office (2010) *Drug Strategy 2010, Reducing Demand Restricting Supply, Building Recovery: Supporting People to Live a Drug-Free Life.* London: HMSO.

Home Office (2012) *Statistical News Release: Drug Misuse Declared Findings from the 2011/12 Crime Survey for England and Wales.* London: HMSO.

Hong, S.-B., Zalesky, A., Cocchi, L., Fornito, A., Choi, E.-J. (2013) Decreased Functional Brain Connectivity in Adolescents with Internet Addiction. *PLoS ONE* 8 (2): e57831. doi:10.1371/journal.pone.0057831.

House of Commons (2010). *Young People's Sexual Health: The National Chlamydia Screening Programme: Seventh Report 2009 – 2010.* London: The Stationery Office Limited.

Hubley, J. and Copeman, J. (2008) *Practical Health Promotion.* Cambridge: Polity Press.

Hughes, B., Russell, R. and Paterson, K. (2005) Nothing to be had 'off the peg': Consumption, identity and the immobilization of young disabled people. *Disability & Society.* 20 (1), 3–17.

Ingham, R. (2005) 'We didn't cover that in school': education against pleasure or education for pleasure? *Sex Education,* 5 (4), 375–388.

Innovation with Substance and Southampton Healthy Schools (2011). *Drug Education Resource Pack: A Guide to Drug Awareness.* IWS & Southampton Healthy Schools.

Ipsos MORI Social Research Institute in association with Nairn, A. (2011) *Children's Well-Being in the UK, Sweden and Spain: The Role of Inequality and Materialism. A Qualitative Study.* London: Ipsos MORI.

Jackson, G. (2005) Cybernetic children: How technologies change and constrain the developing mind. In N. Radcliffe and C. Newnes (eds) *Making and Breaking Children's Lives.* Ross-on-Wye: PCCS Books, pp. 90–105.

Jackson, L. (2002) *Freaks, Geeks and Asperger Syndrome: A User Guide to Adolescence.* London: Jessica Kingsley Publishers.

James, O. (2007) *Affluenza: How to Be Successful and Stay Sane.* London: Vermillion.

Jay, A. (2014) *Independent Inquiry into Child Sexual Exploitation in Rotherham 1997-2013.* Rotherham Metropolitan Borough Council.

Kaner, E. F. et al. (2007) Effectiveness of brief alcohol interventions in primary care populations. *Cochrane Database of Systematic Reviews.* 2.

Kaufman, R. and The Option Institute and Fellowship (2014) *Autism Breakthrough.* New York: St Martin's Press.

Kendel, D. B. Epidemiological & psychosocial perspectives on adolescent drug use. *Journal of American Academic Clinical Psychiatry.* 21, 328–347.

Kenkel, D., Mathios, A. D. and Pacula, R. L. (2001) Economics of youth drug use, addiction and gateway effects. *Addiction.* 96, 151–164.

King, M. and Bearman, P. (2009) Diagnostic change and increased prevalence in autism. *International Journal of Epidemiology*, 38, 1224–1234.

Kirby, D. et al. (2002) The impact of schools and school programs on adolescent sexual behaviour. *The Journal of Sex Research.* 39 (1), 27–33.

Kirby, D. (2009) What have we learnt? What works, what doesn't and ways forward: international evidence. In A. Martinez (ed.) *Celebrating Sex and Relationships Education.* London: National Children's Bureau, pp. 7–16.

Konner, M. (1982) *The Tangled Wing: Biological Constraints on the Human Spirit.* London: Penguin Books.

Konner, M. (1991) *Childhood.* London: Little, Brown and Company.

Konner, M. (2010) *The Evolution of Childhood: Relationships, Emotion, Mind.* London: The Belnap Press of Harvard University Press.

Kroger, J. (2004) *Identity in Adolescence.* London: Routledge.

Kutscher, M. (2007) *Kids in the Syndrome Mix of ADHD, LD, Asperger's, Tourette's, Bipolar, and More!* London: Jessica Kingsley Publishers.

Lansley, A. (2010) *A New Approach to Public Health.* UK Faculty of Public Health Conference, 7 July 2010.

Leach, P. (2010) *Your Baby and Child: From Birth to Age Five.* New York: Alfred A. Knopf.

Lemer, C. (2012). *Annual Report of the Chief Medical Officer 2012: Our Children Deserve Better.* London: HMSO.

Leyshon, M. (2011) *New Media: New Problem? Alcohol, Young People and the Internet.* London: Alcohol Concern.

Linn, S. (2004) *Consuming Kids: The Hostile Takeover of Childhood.* New York: New Press.

Livingstone, S., Haddon, L., Gorzig, A. and Olafsson, K. (2011) *EU Kids OnLine Report.* London: LSE/EU Commission.

Louv, R. (2010) *Last Child in the Woods: Saving Our Children from Nature-Deficit Disorder.* London: Atlantic Books.

Lovell, R. and Roe, J. (2009) Physical and Mental Health Benefits of Participation in Forest Schools. *Countryside Recreation Network.* 17 (1), 20–23.

Lynch, J. and Blake, S. (2004) *Sex, Alcohol and Other Drugs: Exploring the Links in Young People's Lives.* London: National Children's Bureau with the Sex Education Forum and the Drug Education Forum.

Mansfield, K. (1977) in C.K. Stead (ed.) *The Letters and Journals of Katherine Mansfield: A Selection.* Harmondsworth: Penguin.

Mattingley, B. and Harry, R. (2008) Mentro Allan: Some of the stuff we've learnt so far... *Countryside Recreation Network.* 16 (2), 13–17.

Maudsley, M. (2007) *Factsheet No 10: Children's Play in Natural Environments.* London: Children's Play Information Service.

McCoglan, M., Campbell, A. and Marshall, J. (2013) Safeguarding children and child protection. In B. Littlechild and R. Smith (eds) *A Handbook of Interprofessional Practice in the Human Services.* London: Pearson, pp. 117–130.

Mentor: Thinking Prevention. (Jan 2013) Making a public health case for investing in prevention and early intervention initiatives to tackle substance misuse. www.mentoruk.org.uk/publichealth (Accessed 22/05/13).

Middleton, K. (2007) *Eating Disorders: The Path to Recovery.* Oxford: Lion.

Millen, J. V., Irwin, A. and Kim, J. Y. (2000) Introduction: What is growing? Who is dying? In J. Y. Kim, J. V. Millen, A. Irwin and J. Gershman (eds) *Dying for Growth: Global Inequality and the Health of the Poor.* Cambridge, MA: Common Courage Press, pp. 3–10.

MIND (2006) *Ecotherapy: The Green Agenda for Mental Health.* London: Mind Publications.

Mooney, A., Owen, C. and Statham, J. (2008) *Disabled Children: Numbers, Characteristics and Local Service Provision.* London: Thomas Coren Research Institute, University of London/Department of Children and Families.

Moran, P. et al. (2012) The natural history of self-harm from adolescence to young adulthood: A population based cohort study. *The Lancet.* 379 (9812), 236–243.

Moretti, M. and Craig, S. (2013) Maternal versus paternal physical and emotional abuse, affect regulation and risk for depression from adolescence to early adulthood. *Child Abuse & Neglect.* 37 (1), 4–13.

Morris, J. (2002) *Moving into Adulthood.* York: Joseph Rowntree Foundation.

Moss, S. (2012) *Natural Childhood.* London: National Trust.

Moyer, A., Finney, J. W., Swearingen, C. E. and Vergun, P. (2002) Brief interventions for alcohol problems: A meta-analytic review of controlled investigations in treatment-seeking and non-treatment-seeking populations. *Addiction.* 97 (3), 279–292.

Muncie, J. (2014) *Youth and Crime* (4th edition). London: Sage.

Nesse, M. and Williams, G. (1995) *Evolution and Healing: The New Science of Darwinian Medicine.* London: Weidenfeld and Nicolson.

Newman, T. (2004) *What Works in Building Resilience.* Essex: Barnardo's.

Newnes, C. and Radcliffe, N. (eds) (2005) *Making and Breaking Children's Lives.* Ross-on-Wye: PCCS Books.

NHS Information Centre (2010) *Smoking, Drinking and Drug Use among Young People in England: Findings by Region, 2006 – 2008.* Leeds: NCSR & NFER.

NHS (2011) *Statistics on Alcohol: England, 2011 [NS].* Leeds: NHS Information Centre.

NHS, NCSR and NFER (2010) Smoking, Drinking and Drug Use among Young People in England: Findings by Region, *2006-2008. A survey carried out for the NHS Information Centre by NCSR and the NFER.* Leeds: NHS, NCSR and NFER.

NHS National Treatment Agency for Substance Misuse (2005) Tier 4 drug treatment in England: Summary of inpatient provision and needs assessment. www.nta.nhs.uk (Accessed 28/04/16).

NHS National Treatment Agency for Substance Misuse (2010) Substance misuse among young people: the data for 2009–2010. www.nta.nhs.uk (Accessed 28/04/16).

NHS National Treatment Agency for Substance Misuse (2012). *Drug Use Is Declining, More Drug Users Are Recovering. The Original Pool of Heroin and Crack Addicts Is Shrinking. Even so, Plenty of Work Remains to Be Done... Drug Treatment 2012 Progress Made, Challenges Ahead.* London: NHS.

NICE (2004) *Eating Disorders in over 8s: Management.* NICE Guidelines [CG9] January 2004

NICE (2007a) *Interventions to Reduce Substance Misuse Amongst Vulnerable Young People.* London: NICE Public Health Guidance.

NICE (2007b) Quick reference guide: Interventions used to reduce substance misuse among vulnerable young people. www.nice.org.uk/nicemedia/live/11379/41662/41662.pdf (Accessed 23/03/14).

NICE Guidelines [PH14] School based interventions to prevent smoking uptake among children and young people. Evidence Update April 2013.

O'Connor, B. (2003) *Handbook of Solution Focused Therapy.* London: Sage.

Oetting, E. R., Deffenbacher, J. L. and Donnermeyer, J. F. (1998) Primary socialization theory. The role played by personal traits in the etiology of drug use and deviance. *Substance Use and Misuse.* 33 (6).

Oliver, M. (1993) *What's So Wonderful about Walking?* Inaugural Professorial Lecture at University of Greenwich. Leeds: Disability Research Unit.

Oliver, M. (1996) *Understanding Disability: From Theory to Practice.* Basingstoke: Palgrave Macmillan.

OFSTED (2013) *PSHE: Not Yet Good Enough.* London: HMSO.

Ogersby, B. (1998) *Youth in Britain since 1945.* London: Routledge.

Palmer, S. (2006) *Toxic Childhood: How the Modern World Is Damaging Our Children and What We Can Do about It.* London: Orion.

Palmer, S. (2012) *De toxing Childhood.* Conference Presentation. Early Childhood Action Conference: University of Winchester.

Papadopoulos, L. (2011) *Sexualisation of Young People Review.* London: HMSO.

Papadopoulos, L. (2014) *Whose Life Is It Anyway: Living through Your 20s on Your Own Terms.* London: Piatkus.

Patton, G., Coffey, C., Cappa, C. M. and Currie, D. (2012) Health of the world's adolescents: A synthesis of internationally comparable data. *The Lancet.* 379, 1641–1652.

Phoenix, A. (2005) Young consumers. In S. Ding and K. Littleton. *Children's Personal and Social Development.* Open University Press, pp. 221–256.

Pretty, J., Hine, R. and Peacock, J. (2006) Green Exercise: The benefits of activities in green places. *The Biologist.* 53 (3), 142–148.

Pretty, J. et al. (2009) *Nature, Childhood, Health and Life Pathways.* Interdisciplinary Centre for Environment and Society (iCES) Occasional Paper 2009-2: University of Essex.

Priestly, M. (2013) Generating debates: Why we need a life-course approach to disability issues. In J. Swain, S. French, C. Barnes and C. Thomas. (eds) *Disabling Barriers: Enabling Environments* (3rd edition). London: Sage, pp.99–106.

Porter, D. (1999) *Health, Civilisation and the State: A History of Public Health from Ancient to Modern Times.* London: Routledge.

Powell, P., Spears, K. and Rebori, M. (2010) *What Is Obesogenic Environment.* University of Nevada Cooperative Extension.

PSHE Association, Brook, Sex Education Forum (2014) *Sex and Relationships Education (SRE) for the 21st Century New Supplementary Advice.* London: NCB.

Pudney, S. (2002) *The Road to Ruin? Sequences of Initiation into Drug Use and Offending by Young People in Britain.* London: Home Office Research, Development and Statistics Directorate.

Public Health England/AYPH (2013) *Key Data on Adolescence 2013: The Latest Information and Statistics about Young People Today.* London: PHE/AYPH.

Public Health England/AYPH (2014) *Improving Young People's Health: A Framework for Public Health.* London: PHE/AYPH.

Public Health England (2015) *New Evidence Review of Measures to Reduce Sugar Consumption.* London: PHE.

Pycroft, A. (2010) *Understanding & Working with Substance Misusers.* London: Sage.

Quarmby, K. (2011) *Scapegoat: Why We Are Failing Disabled People.* London: Portobello Books.

Ramachandran, V. S. (2011) *The Tell-Tale Brain: Unlocking the Mystery of Human Nature.* London: William Heinemann.

Review of Sex & Relationships Education – A report by the external steering group (2008) http://webarchive.nationalarchives.gov.uk/20130401151715/https://www.education.gov.uk/publications/eOrderingDownload/SRE-Review-2008.pdf (Accessed 29/03/14).

Rikwood, S., Deane, F., Wilson, C. and Ciarrochi, J. (2005) Young people's help-seeking for mental health problems. *Australian e-Journal for the Advancement of Mental Health, (supplement).* http://ro.uow.edu.au/cgi/viewcontent.cgi?article=3159&context=hbs papers (Accessed 28/04/16).

Roberts, H. (2012) *What Works in Reducing Inequalities in Child Health* (2nd edition). Bristol: Policy Press.

Roberts, R., O'Connor, T. G., Dunn, J. and Golding, J. (2004) The effects of child sexual abuse in later family life: Mental health, parenting and adjustment of offspring. *Child Abuse & Neglect.* 28 (5), 525–545.

Rogers, C. (1996) *The Carl Rogers Reader.* London: Constable.

Romano M., Osborne, L. A., Truzoli, R. and Reed, P. (2013) Differential psychological impact of internet exposure on internet addicts. *PLoS ONE* 8 (2), e55162. doi:10.1371/journal.pone.0055162.

Rutter, M. (1987) Psychosocial resilience and protective mechanisms. *American Journal of Orthopsychiatry.* 57, 316–331.

Selikowitz, M. (2004) *Dyslexia and Other Learning Difficulties: The Facts.* Oxford: Oxford University Press.

Sigman, A. (2007) Visual voodoo: The biological impact of watching television. *The Biologist.* 54 (1), 12–17.

Seligman, M. (2007) *Authentic Happiness: Using the New Positive Psychology to Realize Your Potential for Lasting Fulfillment.* London: Nicholas Brealey Publishing.

Seligman, M. (2008) Positive health. *Applied Psychology: An International Review.* 57, 3–18.

Sigman, A. (2011) *Alcohol Nation: How to Protect Our Children from Today's Drinking culture:* London: Piatkus.

Silberman, S. (2015) *Neurotribes: The Legacy of Autism and How to Think Smarter about People Who Think Differently.* London: Allen & Unwin.

Simmons, R. and Blyth, D. (1987) *Moving into Adolescence: The Impact of Pubertal Change and School Context.* New York: Aldine de Gruyter.

Smith, T. (1993) Influence of socioeconomic factors on attaining targets for reducing teenage pregnancies. *British Medical Journal.* 306, 1232–1235.

Snyder, G. (1961) Buddhist Anarchism. www.purifymind.com/Anarchism.htm (Accessed 28/04/16).

Sourander, A., Multimaki, P. and Santalahti, P. (2004) Mental health service use among 18-year-old boys: A prospective 10 year follow-up study. *Journal of the American Academy of Child and Adolescent Psychiatry.* 43 (10), 1150–1158.

Starkey, F. et al. (2009) Identifying influential young people to undertake peer-led health promotion: The example of a Stop Smoking in Schools Trial (ASSIST). *Health Education Research.* 24 (6), 977–988.

Sten, L., Van Den Berg, A. and De Groot, M. (2013) Environmental psychology: History, scope, methods. In L. Sten, A. Van Den Berg and M. De Groot (eds) *Environmental Psychology: An Introduction.* Chichester: BPS Blackwell.

Stengard, E. and Appelqvist-Schmidlechner, K. (2010) *Mental Health Promotion in Young People – An Investment for the Future.* Copenhagen: WHO Europe.

Strelitz, J. (2013) Chapter 3: The economic case for a shift to prevention. In the Chief Medical Officer's Report. *Prevention Pays: Our Children Deserve Better.* London: Department of Health.

Stott, R. (2000) *The Ecology of Health.* Dartington: Green Books/Schumacher Society.

Sunstein, C. R. (2008) Adolescent risk-taking and social meaning: A commentary. *Developmental Review.* 28, 145–152.

Telegraph (27 May 2011) Alcohol-related hospital admissions top one million. http://www.telegraph.co.uk/news/health/news/8538849/Alcohol-related-hospital-admissions-top-one-million.html (Accessed 18/03/14).

Timimi, S. and Radcliffe, N. (2005) The rise and rise of ADHD. In C. Newnes and N. Radcliffe (eds) *Making and Breaking Children's Lives.* Ross-on-Wye: PCCS Books, pp. 63–70.

Tisdall, K. (2001) Failing to make transition? Theorizing the 'transition to adulthood for young disabled people. In M. Priestly (ed.) *Disability and the Life Course: Global Perspectives.* Cambridge: Cambridge University Press, pp. 167–178.

Thane, P. (1996) *Foundations of the Welfare State.* London: Longman.

The Children's Act (2004) London: HMSO.

The Children's Society (2012) *Good Childhood Report: A Review of Our Children's Well-Being.* Leeds: The Children's Society.

The Children's Society (2012) *Good Childhood Report: A Report for Decision Makers in Parliament, Central Government and Local Areas.* Leeds: The Children's Society.

The Drug Education Forum (2016) *The principles of good drug education.* http://mentor-adepis.org/the-principles-of-good-drug-education (Accessed 28/04/16).

The Guardian (2013) Hospital admissions linked to alcohol rise to more than a million in year. http://www.theguardian.com/society/2013/may/30/hospital-admissions-alcohol-million-year (Accessed 12 August 2013).

The Safe Network (2013) Annual Cyber-Bullying Survey. Ditch the Label. www.schools-out.org.uk (Accessed 28/04/16).

The Observer (2008) Drugs in literature: A brief history. www.theguardian.com/society/2008/nov/16/drugs-history-literature (Accessed 23/03/14).

Thio, A. (1975) A critical look at Merton's Anomie Theory. *The Pacific Sociological Review.* 18 (2), 139–158.

Thurstone, C. (2013) *Essential Nursing Care for Children and Young People: Theory, Policy and Practice.* London: Routledge.

Tither, J. and Ellis, B. (2008) Impact of fathers on daughters' age at menarche: A genetically and environmentally controlled sibling study. *Developmental Psychology.* 44 (5),1409–1420.

Treffert, D. A. (2010) *Islands of Genius: The Bountiful Mind of the Autistic, Acquired and Sudden Savant.* London: Jessica Kingsley Publishers.

Turkle, S. (2010) *Alone Together: Why We Expect More from Technology and Less from Each Other.* New York: Basic Books.

UK Youth Parliament (2007) *SRE: Are You Getting It?* London: UK Youth Parliament.

Ungar, M. et al. (2013) Patterns of service use, individual and contextual risk factors, and resilience among adolescents using multiple psychosocial services. *Child Abuse & Neglect.* 13 (2–3), 150–159.

UNICEF/WHO (2007) *Child Poverty in Perspective: An Overview of Child Well-Being in Rich Countries. A Comprehensive Assessment of the Lives and Well-Being of Children and Adolescents in the Economically Advanced Nations.* Florence: Innocenti Research Centre, UNICEF.

UNICEF (2011) *The State of the World's Children 2011: Adolescence: An Age of Opportunity.* New York: UNICEF.

Urry, J. (1990) *The Tourist Gaze.* London: Sage.

Van den Berg, A., Joyce, Y. and de Vries, S. (2013) Health benefits of nature. In L. Steg et al. (eds) *Environmental Psychology: An Introduction.* Oxford: Blackwell/British Psychological Society Textbooks, pp. 47–56.

Viner, R. (2012) Life stage: Adolescence. In *Annual Report of the Chief Medical Officer 2012, Our Children Deserve Better: Prevention Pays.* London: HMSO.

Vostanis, P. (2007) *Mental Health and Mental Disorders.* J. Coleman and A. Hagell (eds) *Adolescence, Risk and Resilience: Against the Odds.* Chichester: John Wiley & Sons, pp. 89–106.

Watson, M. (2008) Catch a Kid and Change a Life. *Countryside Recreation Network.* 16 (2), 3–5.

Weare, K. (2005) Taking a positive, holistic, approach to the mental and emotional health and well-being of children and young people. In C. Newnes and N. Radcliffe (eds) *Making and Breaking Children's Lives.* Ross-on-Wye: PCCS Books. pp. 115–122.

Wilk, A. I. et al. (1997) Meta-analysis of randomised control trials heavy alcohol drinkers. *Archives of Internal Medicine.* 12, 274–283.

Wilkinson, R. and Pickett, K. (2010) *The Spirit Level: Why Equality Is Better for Everyone.* London: Penguin.

Williams, R. (1995) *NHS Health Advisory Review on Child and Adolescent Mental Health Services.* London: HMSO.

Wilson, E. O. (2012) *The Social Conquest of Earth.* New York: Liveright Publishing.

Wolfe, N. (2011) *The Viral Storm: The Dawn of a New Pandemic Age.* London: Allen Lane Books.

Wolfensberger, W. (1989) Human service policies: The rhetoric versus the reality. In L. Barton (ed.) *Disability and Dependence.* Lewes: Falmer, pp. 23–40.

World Health Organization (1984) Health Promotion: A WHO discussion document on the concepts and principles. Reprinted in: *Journal of the Institute of Health Education.* 23 (1), 1985.

World Health Organization (1986) *The Ottawa Charter for Health Promotion.* Geneva: WHO.

World Health Organization (2001) *The World Mental Health Report 2001. Mental Health: New Understanding, New Hope.* Geneva: WHO.

World Health Organization (2006) *Defining Sexual Health – Report of a Technical Consultation on Sexual Health 28–31 January 2002,* Geneva: WHO.

World Health Organization (2007) *International Classification of Functioning Disability and Health – Children and Young People.* Geneva: WHO.

Young Minds (2013) Young Carers. www.youngminds.org.uk (Accessed 28/04/16).

Youth Access (2013) *Picking Up the Pieces: Results of a Survey on the State of Young People's Advice, Counselling and Support Services.* London: Young People's Health Partnership.

Youth Media Agency (2012) *Submission to Levenson Inquiry: Children, Young People and the UK Press.* London: Youth Media Agency.

Yuan, K. et al. (2011) Microstructure abnormalities in adolescents with internet addiction disorder. *PLoS ONE* 6 (6), e20708. doi:10.1371/journal.pone.0020708.

INDEX